WHAT PEOPLE ARE S

DEAR POPPYSEED

Written in a personable and instantly engaging way one minute you find yourself smiling, nodding your head in agreement and the next weeping at the sheer beauty of the heartfelt letters Alice writes to her unborn child. Simply the most divine pregnancy book you will ever read.
Charlie Plunkett author of *The True Diary of a Mum-to be and Baby's First Year* www.charlieplunkett.co.uk

Dear Poppyseed is a poignant account of pregnancy that manages to be both grounded and spiritual. Reading it evoked so many memories of my own three pregnancies and made me long to feel those precious first days of knowing and glowing once more. Alice successfully captures the universal emotions of motherhood through this intimate diary
Lucy Pearce author *Moods of Motherhood* and *Moon Time: a guide to celebrating your menstrual cycle.* Contributing editor JUNO magazine.

Poppyseed is a refreshing combination of being light hearted, informative, honest and deep. It touched my heart immediately, and is a must for anyone who is pregnant or thinking of having children. Bonding begins in the womb and this book is a wonderful example of how to welcome and connect lovingly to your baby from the earliest moments. I encourage all parents to follow in Alice's footsteps and write a pregnancy diary, liberally interspersed with love letters to their own 'poppyseed'.
Kitty Hagenbach child & parent psychotherapist – Co founder of Babies Know www.babiesknow.com

As a man I find the story insightful and very moving on occasions. I love the depth of honesty and attention to detail that is both fascinating and also makes me squirm. I especially enjoyed the transformations occurred in all three of you as the birth draws nearer and nearer, and how the birth took so much longer than expected. The soulful mother has to trust her daughter to emerge when she needs and wants to, not when the doctors told her it might happen.
Nick Clements Author of *The New Ages of Men* and *Alpha Wolf*

'Any woman who wishes to have a soulful pregnancy and birth cannot afford to be without this book! Written with honesty, humor; every emotion and physical symptom rings true in a way I haven't read before in a pregnancy book. Intrinsically, this is book about balance. Balance between the physical and spiritual, the needs of the mum and the baby, the alternative and the medical. It shows that in all ways all of these can be in harmony, if approached in a soulful and mindful way.
I laughed out loud, I worried with her and I supported her through her birth even though I knew that her baby had been born. This shows how caught up I was in this wonderful book!'
Colette Brown author of *Menopause, A Natural and Spiritual Journey*

Writing this through tears! I feel as though I have just given birth, without the grunting. What an amazing book this is. Written in an honest way that shares the happiness, funniness and anxiety of the whole 'growing a baby' process. Describing it as an emotional roller coaster doesn't come close. My advice: if you're pregnant, want to be, have/haven't been, or any combination of nature that may or may not involve having a baby, read this book. You'll be sharing the experience with Alice, James, the bunnies and the cats. Dear Poppyseed, I love you
Barbara Ford Hammond author of *The Psychic Way*

'I've not yet had to read a book about pregnancy, babies or being a momma and guess what? After reading Poppyseed, I'm never going to have to read another, because this is the most beautiful, honest and heart-filled book about the journey to mummahood you'll ever read. Alice shares candidly her thoughts, feelings and experiences - everything from nipples that feel like they're on fire, to the sweet declarations of love to Poppyseed - I laughed out loud, I cried and I feel better knowing that if ever I'm blessed to experience mummahood, Alice has totally got my back!'
Lisa Clark author of *SASSY: The Go-for-it Girl's Guide to Becoming Mistress of Your Destiny*

Many books have been written on impending motherhood, but none truly 'get' how a mother to be feels in preparation for bringing baby into the world. All the fears, the excitement, the preparation for birth itself, is covered here - This book is simply wonderful, you will feel like Alice is holding your hand whilst you go through the journey yourself. And, perhaps it will inspire you to write something similar for your own child - a true gift, for both of you!
Anna Rodgers author of *How to thrive in our toxic world - a guide to health, beauty, parenting and conscious living*

Dear Poppyseed is the personal journey of a mother during pregnancy. It's an honest account of her vulnerabilities, hopes, insecurities, dreams and visions as a mother-to-be.

Alice Grist's pregnancy journal reminds us all that parenting is a rich world with so much potential for growth, even before the baby arrives in our arms. Mothers around the world will feel united at the common threads we share on this path of pregnancy. Mother and child will look back upon this journal and see it as an integral part of their lives; a record of possibility scribed from the open heart of a beautiful and inspired mother. By sharing this intimate book, other parents will feel supported

and inspired during their pregnancies.
Veronika Sophia Robinson Author and Founder / Editor of *The Mother Magazine*

Dear Poppyseed

A Soulful Momma's Pregnancy Journey

Dear Poppyseed

A Soulful Momma's Pregnancy Journey

Alice Grist

SOUL Rocks

Winchester, UK
Washington, USA

First published by Soul Rocks Books, 2013
Soul Rocks Books is an imprint of John Hunt Publishing Ltd., Laurel House, Station Approach,
Alresford, Hants, SO24 9JH, UK
office1@jhpbooks.net
www.johnhuntpublishing.com
www.soulrocks-books.com

For distributor details and how to order please visit the 'Ordering' section on our website.

ISBN: 978 1 78099 647 9

A CIP catalogue record for this book is available from the British Library.

Design: Stuart Davies

Printed in the USA by Edwards Brothers Malloy

For my Poppyseed…

About the Author

Alice Grist is the author of *The High Heeled Guide to Enlightenment* and *The High Heeled Guide to Spiritual Living* (Prediction Magazine Best Book Award 2012). This, *Dear Poppyseed, A Soulful Momma's Pregnancy Journal,* is her third book.

Alice contributes articles to a number of magazines online and in print. She is the imprint publisher of Soul Rocks books, publishing soulful, edgy and entertaining writings for the next generation.

She lives with her husband James, their two cats, and of course, her little Poppyseed…

Follow Alice's continued journey as a Soulful Momma here: www.alicegrist.co.uk

Introduction

I'll keep this brief. This book is the diary of my pregnancy. If you know my work you will know I have spent some years on a spiritual path, which I have explored and written about with gusto. Two books down the line, and the next challenge was an altogether more human and earthy one. Pregnancy.

This diary is taken from my actual pen and paper diary that I wrote for myself and for my unborn baby. It is a record of what went on physically, emotionally, mentally and spiritually during the gestation period. I hope that this very real account will be a good little read for any woman who is, wants to be, or has ever been pregnant. Whether she is soulful, spiritual or entirely neither, this book reveals the fantastic wonderful highs and the nauseous, gaseous lows of a first time momma who is trying her hardest to do things with a pinch of soul.

This needs no more explaining. I had a beautiful little baby and here is my deeply personal insight on how it happened...

Dear Poppyseed,

I found out I was pregnant with you on the day of a full moon. Before I realized you were with me, I had done my usual ritual of taking a guidance card for the day. It said upon it 'Full Moon – Completion', the card spoke in fancy terms of gestation, something brewing, coming to fruition. I didn't know it was you. And that of course is not even the beginning, it never is.

We planned you in a relaxed kind of way. Your Dad and I, we never plan anything properly. We don't make lists or draw up laborious maps of our life. We make up our minds and then things happen. We are haphazard, blundering perhaps, but so far our blunders tend to turn to gold. We married in Vegas after eight years, and after ten years we decided to have a go and see if you wanted to come along. On our first month of an open invite, you accepted. I feel very honored that you were so quick to respond.

As for the other events that precipitated your arrival, well this is where you find out what a soppy hippy your Mom is. Firstly, I felt you implant in me. I was driving to see your Great Grandma Grist for her 90th Birthday and I experienced what seemed like a pencil drawing something deep inside me. I am sure this was you settling yourself in. I asked my angels and guides for a sign, and at that moment, a car went by with a sign on the window that said 'little person on board'. What could I do, I smiled!

Later that night the cause of my hippy ways, your Pagan Grandpa Tony and I, were reading our tarot cards and quite clearly you were there. Up came the image of a little tiny baby, nestled in an egg, and held carefully in a Woman's arms. This deeply meaningful card glared up from the table right into my heart. The card was The Moon, it seems you are my little ray of Luna Light. The synchronicities thus far suggest loudly to me that you and me, my little love, are meant to be. I know already that you are the biggest piece of my soulful and personal growth, and come hell or high water, I will do my best.

Before I had even had a pregnancy test we had chosen your

name. In giving you a name, I guessed that you were inside me. But I didn't want to admit it for fear I was wrong. I pondered on the thought that maybe this baby naming game was part of some cruel self-inflicted fantasy. Your Dad and I had literally only just started trying to get pregnant. But something felt different. I was averse to making plans for my birthday – which is so very unlike me! I knew that there was a very good chance I would not be celebrating with champagne. I avoided the gym too – perhaps not so unusual - but I had a feeling that jumping about and getting sweaty was not what my body needed right now. So I obeyed these inner instincts. Already you have me digging deeper. Listening to my intuition more than ever.

The following weekend I attended my first class of a spiritual based therapy course that I had signed up to for the next ten months. I knew when I signed up to this course that it might coincide with you. Whilst this might be a problem in terms of attendance in my late stages of pregnancy, it feels right. I am sure that what I learn here is preparing some foundations, helping me firm up how I see the world, putting it into a context that will suit us.

On this course I went on a Shamanic Journey – a spiritual meditation type adventure - to meet my guiding power animals. So to the beat of a drum, I let my mind voyage past imagination and into a place where things apparently started to happen of their own accord. In this inner vision, I met my animal and he took me to a man. A man I believe was you, or your guide. Either way he was linked to my future child, that much I was certain of. He too had an animal. Our animals lit up the jungle with loud roars and as I recognized a miracle I felt your spirit move into me. This was undeniable and powerful. I couldn't speak for a while after. I was dumbstruck, choking on emotion and it was beautiful. You are beautiful. I know your spirit is with me now.

The night of meeting you in the shamanic journey, I took you to a cage fight. The least appropriate place for an unborn child, but still, life is life and people fight in cages. So what. Live and let live. Your Dad's friend was in his first fight, and the atmosphere was brutally male. Sadly our guy lost, but he's a fighter, much like you will be I am sure. Someone who will always take life's blows and come back wiser, confident, stronger, with an inner faith in your abilities.

The next day, feeling very bloated and as though my period was due, I decided to do the test to see if I was pregnant. I was scared that I was living out of my imagination, and didn't want to be dreadfully disappointed when my period came. But of course, two tests later and I was as red as a beetroot, on the phone to your Dad, telling him that I was pregnant. I then had the longest phone call in my life to a client about something or other, before I could get off and tell our friends and family. Two more tests later and you are very much confirmed.

We are all very excited, all your new family. Your Dad and me are transformed already. He even put the pizza in the oven last night. He burnt it, but he put it in the oven. Trust me, this is a jaw dropping change. As I type he is making himself a bacon sandwich, I am amazed at his newfound ability to prepare food without resorting to the microwave.

Daddy warns me not to feign symptoms or to become a helpless pregnant wreck, but if I try to do something for myself he rushes to my side and takes over. He has been kissing my head an awful lot. I love it, but I think deep down he is really kissing you. We just got back from the doctors and even though they talk in fearful terms of what to do, what not to do, serious tests, I have a quiet faith that all will be well.

I hope you don't mind me writing to you, and about you. The last thing I had to say in my previous book was I'm spiritual, what next? Now I have a more important question, I'm pregnant; this trumps everything, what next now? I want to give you the best and handle this in the most soulful way a person possibly can. I won't ask you to be like me, but I will feed your soul in every way I can. The next eight months is an adventure of all of that. A big mish mash amalgamation of bodily matters, spiritual concerns, physical craziness, and a whole lot of love.

I'll be really honest now. I know nothing about what comes next. Right now you are the size of a poppyseed and I can still fit in my skinny jeans. The only thing I do know is, that you are loved unconditionally now and forevermore.

Love, from your Mum

So it seems I'm Pregnant…

I am four weeks pregnant but to my actual official knowledge it's only been a week. In spite of this, I have suffered backache pretty much since conception, so I had an inkling…

Apparently, the next two months represent the most dangerous time of pregnancy. And so everything changes. Overnight. It's not only the danger that forces change. It's the hope, the joy, the excitement, the sudden desire to put myself first, but only because there is a little teensy weensy baby growing inside me.

Within seconds my relationship to everything has vastly altered. My marriage has apparently become deeply more significant. There is love beyond love, and all those little niggly arguments, well, they have vanished (more or less and of course I'll keep you updated). Friendships seem different as my socializing options instantly minimize. Some people want to talk baby, some don't. Both options are fine. More often than not, I have no choice. I try to talk book, and people talk baby back. I give up. This is all about the baby, a language I am only just learning to speak. Please let's not get so far as nappies yet. I'm still coping with immediately expanding boobs and random exhaustion. Conversations and thoughts of nappies, vaginal stitches and bladder weakness can all wait.

My understanding of biology is broadening as I set foot on the initial weeks of baby development. Who knew all the tiny miracles that occur everyday to make up the miracle that is my first child? There is already a strain on myself as I aim to do my best, but constantly feel I could be doing more…I should not have eaten those crisps…so make vegetable soup to compensate. I'm chasing my tail, and my tailbone is actually aching as my body adapts to the pains of growing a little one.

Something that really interests me, and the partial reason for this diary, is the spiritual and personal changes that I presume will occur in my life. I say 'presume' because for the past few years I have been indulging in my own spiritual path, wallowing in it, bathing in it, and loving it. I have tried to be soulfulness personified. I am happy to report that because of these efforts I have become a better person. I'm not blowing my own trumpet, it's true. Nor am I perfect, but I am better. I'm happier and saner than I was several years ago. A spiritual path has been like a massive dose of therapeutic self-help.

So now that I have contentedly found myself, what will this trip of pregnancy and parenthood bring to my life? Will it be soulful, or am I headed onto a wholly more physical plane whereby all that matters is what I can see and wrap my arms around?

I spoke strongly in my last book, *The High Heeled Guide to Spiritual Living*, that all things are spiritual, and so I believe that this pregnancy, this giving of life, this giving of myself to another person, is as spiritual as it gets. If indeed this parent-to-be trip does turn out to be deeply soulful, will that be because of an expanding waistline or inspite of it? I'm thinking, in this early stage that it may be because of it. If I can embrace all that pregnancy brings, the gritty, earthy, primal nature of it, then maybe I will have found all I will ever need. And until I shave my head and move to Nepal, this could be as spiritual as it ever gets. Whilst child abandonment may have been good enough for the

Buddha (who left his wife and child to pursue enlightenment) it's a step too far for little old me. So with total abandon, I embrace whatever happens next.

I'm intrigued to see how I might combine my soulful inclinations with the very biological inclinations of pregnancy? Well happily, I have come to terms with the fact that human life is the most important thing we have on our plates right now. We are not here to float off into some divine mist, not yet. We are not above and beyond the carnal, the physical, the fights and the failures.

And so, as I head into the world of parenting, allowing those very human based activities to take centre stage. Which is a good job because several days into this pregnancy and before I knew I was 'up the duff', I went out and got horribly drunk (I blame the over generous barman). Not a great start. But, a good lesson in self-forgiveness. I'm on the fruit, veggies and pure water from now on of course. As a soulful human, and as a future parent, I suspect I need to occasionally let myself off the hook.

You know that thing spiritual types talk about, giving over, releasing, allowing life to happen, living in the moment, being grateful, and focusing the mind. Well I have a feeling that pregnancy will pretty much force me to embrace those concepts far more deeply than I previously knew possible. How can you know how to release until another being inhabits and takes over your body? How can you be grateful until you realize the joy of ripping yourself open in labor, potentially undergoing mad pain, but yet being ridiculously happy to see the tiny little person who has caused you all that agony?

On paper, pregnancy, childbirth and what comes after, seems to me to be the most soulful undertaking a person can undertake. Lucky for us Women that we have the option! Though I'm sure our partners would argue that they too go through a gritty spiritual mill in supporting us, holding our hands, watching us torn asunder with aches and pains, and that they too find some enlightenment at the end of the deep dark birth canal.

Writing this, I have happily convinced myself. Pregnancy and all that comes after is one sure way to taste a little enlightenment. It's one simple way to find yourself, forget yourself and rise from the ashes anew. It is one way to taste your soul. I may be wrong. I may be right. I may learn something else altogether. Luckily I have eight months ahead to figure this one out. This is the biggest adventure I've ever undertaken and I have a feeling it could lead anywhere.

24th September 2011
It's my birthday! I am a big time birthday girl. I normally harp on about what to do, where to go or what I want for several weeks, nay, months, beforehand. But my birthday only showed up on my mental radar when James started to make mysterious phones calls and come downstairs all giddy saying he's organized something amazing for me. Here I am, on my birthday, writing this diary. Above all other things this pregnancy now takes precedence. Birthdays come and go, but right now there is only one birth day I'm interested in. Who needs gifts when I have that to look forward to! Though of course gifts are appreciated too, and I couldn't guarantee total emotional stability should I not receive any. Such a contradictory thing I am right now!

These past two weeks have been so incredible. Once the romantic pregnancy bubble lifted a little, and life went back to business as usual, the incredible-ness has remained. So whatever irks me or yanks my chain, I am safe in the knowledge that a little something special is going on, and no grumpy colleague, or traffic jam, or afternoon morning sickness can touch it.

It's occurred to me in the past few days how very, very early days this pregnancy is. There have been a couple of moments where I have kidded myself that my being bloated from too much bread, was in fact a growing bump. But following a good nights sleep, said bump has vanished and I am left again with my same old, almost (but never quite been) flat stomach.

There is a certain fear instilled to the early days of pregnancy. I know it's a risky time, but it's hardly base-jumping is it? That said I know people who have lost babies in the early days. I know that horrendous shit can happen, it happens all happens all the time to people who don't deserve it. But this dwelling on fear, on the first twelve weeks as being vital, is oppressive. I have started to dread going to the toilet. Every little twinge is amplified as I half expect to find that I just got my period late and my body has decided I'm not pregnant anymore. Just now I was taking a moderately warm bath, when all of a sudden I awoke from my rested state, jumped out of the bath pronto and went to cool down. All because I had read something worrying about raising the body temperature in saunas, which now remembered, sent me into a dither.

As this is my first baby, I have the luxury of being careful with myself. But what about all those second time mommas who run around after their first child for the first twelve weeks, and still manage to have reasonable pregnancies with healthy babies? What about all those Moms who drink and smoke and eat junk food and have reasonable pregnancies and give birth to healthy babies? Moreover, what about all those crack addicts, who drink too much, sleep rough and sell their bodies, who go on to to have reasonable pregnancies and healthy babies. It does happen. Life is funny like that. Just as there is always the perfect momma who does everything by the book and suffers miscarriage after miscarriage.

Life has a dark and twisted sense of humor. We get what we are given, and we do with it as we can. We can choose to structure our lives, and Vesuvius can then rain down on our heads. The only luxury we have at the end of all this is a little positive thinking. So that, is what I intend to indulge. Quite frankly life is a dangerous game, pregnant or otherwise and happy thoughts are one fabulous way to cope with whatever hurtles our way. If I am very lucky, as can also happen, then happy thoughts can come true.

Of course, at the same time I am heeding all the baby rules, and I'm trying to do my best. I won't drink, I don't smoke, I'll happily take any excuse to avoid the gym and I'm very cool with early nights. I'm not as young as I used to be and I love my bed! I won't allow any fear to consume me. I have to be confident and positive that all will be well.

All things happen for a reason, and if the worst did happen, as it has to many of my friends, then I guess you find a way to dust yourself off and move forward, try again, think happy all over. Easier said than done of course, but essential to a healthy pregnancy and a healthy, sane life. We must think happy thoughts and happiness will result. Again easier said than done, but what is the other option? Sink into despair, rail against god; scream to the skies that life is unfair. Life is unfair. Fact. All we can do is hope and trust and believe that every so often things will go our way. Life will take us where we need to go, with as many pit stops and occasional car crashes as she sees fit.

My soulful inclinations told me I was going to have this baby, and that I must stick to. I can't allow a host of fear factor grossness and the bad experiences of others to impinge on my own little bubble. I can raise my hat to the warnings and do everything I can in my power to take good care, but beyond that, I'm planning for a healthy, happy baby no complications, no worries, and no scares. Like I said, happy thoughts. So for now, my faith is all I've got. Faith, hope and a whole boat load of morning sickness.

Morning sickness – why do they still call it that? That is quite clearly a terrible lie. I have been getting mine in the afternoon. Gosh darn it, why be complicated, let's just call it sickness.

So other than all of those random thoughts, how has my life

actually been? Well last night my darling musician husband James and my best friend Roisin arranged a surprise party for me. Thank goddess someone let it slip mid afternoon, and the surprise was ruined. This was a blessing. I'm a little highly strung right now, and if I was preparing for a night out with my husband ala romantic style, I may not have reacted so well to a big 'surprise' and a vanishing of my Parisian intentions. Ohh la la indeed.

Not that I'm ungrateful. But let's just say I was glad I had the afternoon to adjust to the new plan and to get excited about a night with lovely friends. We arrived half an hour late due to me having a mega nap. I never nap in the day. I can't do it. But this pregnancy malarkey is kicking the hell out of my intentions to stay awake. I now nap like a cat, easily, intensely, purring.

It was lovely to spend a night out feeling normal, totally myself, and not totally consumed with baby banter. Though it was also very lovely to be sat next to a secretly pregnant good mate of mine, Gaynor. We enjoyed our little pregnant lady asides whilst watching the rest of the table getting progressively more drunken! Good food, good friends, good to be out and about and able to be me without feeling little Miss, or Mr, has taken over my mental state completely!

Today my two wifeys came to see me for lunch. The best birthday present being that wifey Reina declared herself to be pregnant too! This was a massive and unexpected happy surprise. Now, the best thing about this is that Reina and I have always joked that we should have kids at the same time. But we didn't actually plan this. Nor did we know the other was trying. It's happened, because we probably always knew deep down that it would do. It's unexpected, but strangely unsurprising. As ever we are running parallel on where we are at in life. So now I have a buddy, as do our future babies.

Everything happens for a reason, and whilst Reina, Gaynor and I have all had our dark times of late, to find we are in this little mama-to-be place together is nothing short of miraculous. If you've read my other books about non-coincidence and things happening for a reason, then apply this here. This is one of those amazing things in life that happens when you are paying no attention. I have baby making soul mates and I'm so happy!

Dear Poppyseed,
You are making me have some really crazy dreams, oh baby of mine. Indeed, it's not fair either that you have put me off chocolate and cake. I never knew such things were possible. You are clearly a powerful soul, and I will take that into account little one when you arrive. I won't mess with you, because anyone with the power to turn me against chocolate and cake is a wizard in the making.

Oh and the whole making me feel sick thing… I can deal with that. It's all good. I'm still in a little bubble of you and so when I feel sick I know it's worth it. Feeling sick is slowly becoming a good thing, who would have thought it! Everything changes through pregnant eyes.

Love you little Poppyseed

Your Momma, Alice

2nd October 2011
A week of contrasts, and a clear indication that trying to be overtly soulful, whilst overcome with the curse of nausea is near impossible. This pregnancy thing is very, very physical. I am in the grasp of my body. My body is overtaking me in ways previously unknown. The tiredness too, it tends to sneak up out of nowhere. It renders plans of baby related rituals, meditations and spiritual connections less desirable. But as per my usual mantra,

all life is spiritual, even the intense moments of sickness, the fatigue, the moments of weakness where a craving for pizza is satiated tenfold!

Earlier this week, I had a full day of nausea. It was killer. By the end of that day I doubted everything. I was in fear of losing my identity. The nausea rushed through me and I became acutely aware that all things would now be different. It was not just that my body was wracked with an unacceptable sick feeling, but the fact that this would give way to slavish physical devotion to a growing bump and the difficulties that might follow. The child that comes from this will need me like no other, and come darkness or disease I must be there for them – till death us do part. This is big time commitment, the likes of which no marriage would be expected to endure. I feel like the time in my life for resting has gone, I miss it. When I feel very tired, that is a harsh thought. I certainly like to rest.

This tiny Poppyseed embryo is my life. All that came before this is gone, it is dead. In a good moment that is freeing and exhilarating, in a nauseous moment that thought can be terrifying. Perhaps I am letting the nausea get the better of me. Or maybe a new reality is truly dawning and if so I hope I will adjust and accept easily.

The next twenty or so years are fairly well mapped; except it is a land I have never visited. In the past I have created my own map. Our niece Elly even said how bizarre it was that we were having a child because James and I had always done what we wanted, and of course now we cannot. But the positive spin, I realized, was that having a baby was our choice. This was our choice. We did this because we wanted to. What we have lost as a result is part of that choice too. I guess only in my moments of deepest exhaustion does that choice take on a gloomier slant. And the gloomy slant is not a place I am going to dwell. We are on this earth but a few moments and there are no mistakes. This child is a blessing. One that will change everything, but I choose to believe that those changes will be for the best, for the happiest and for the most powerful spiritual learning yet.

I may sound as though I'm being heavy and morose. So let me be clear on one thing. I am ready. I want this child with a passion previously unknown. I have wanted a child because for several years now, something has been missing. And as much as a spiritual philosophy would tell me that what was missing is found only within myself, I also know that as a sociable animal, what was missing was the warmth and learning of a little family. Fact. I am not a monk, or a Nun (been there done that – as a past life regression once showed). It is okay to want more from time to time. I am not craving a fast car, to win the lottery, or a new home. But what I do desire is the communication and life events that come with loving and raising a little person.

I want to bring forth another soul mate, someone with whom I will live, learn and love. I want to commit my time to helping make someone else happy. I desire that experience. I crave it. Even in the potential moments of toddler tantrums and screaming madness, I must always remember that I want this, I need this. This is my life. I have chosen this.

Dear Poppyseed,
The world is a scary place and so many people fail to cope well with it. No one tells you that when you are little. And I guess I won't tell you either, not till you are wise enough and strong enough to understand. In my life I have known many people who are failing to cope, or, maybe not failing, but simply coping in their own very mixed up ways. This is not so unusual. Failure to cope seems to be part of the package on this planet.

The world is a very big ancient place, we come here and after eighteen years or so we have learned a great deal. But what have we really learned, compared to what there is to know? By the time we are adult, we know so very little, relatively speaking. All of us have a set of experiences by which we interpret the world, but whose to say what circumstances represent a true understanding? We are on this planet for two brief seconds, and in thinking we know it, or know how to live well, we are often very much mistaken.

Even the tenants of science or religion, or even Momma's spirituality are only ever based on a faith of some sort. Science has faith in numbers and evidence garnered from that which we can see, from evidence correlated by testing specifics. Religion has faith in what we cannot see and yet it's strength is as pungent in its believers as the certain knowing of their existence. Whatever we think, believe, perceive or know, it is all based within the human senses. These senses, our human brains, are wholly fallible. Basing life around intelligence, understanding or perception may in the future prove to be wholly inaccurate. I believe that we humans know so very little, and this, my dear is why we have periods where we fail to cope. And that is OK. Like I said its part of the package. No one really knows anything… though they will always try to tell you they know everything!

My spiritual take on the world is changing, and that is down to your Dad, he is getting feisty with his philosophy and it's making me care a lot less about the meaning of anything – in a good way. I do know there is something more to life… but beyond that I'm not too specific or fussy. I'm settling nicely into the here and now. I think that maybe that is your influence too, and it's a good, relevant, timely influence.

As a person who has written two spiritual books (and therefore someone who supposedly 'knows') I am sure that it is okay not to know the details of the ever after or indeed of our true spiritual make up. I think anyone who claims to know is either fibbing, power tripping or a tad delusional. I don't care what book you read or which theology you practice, none of us know anything really. We can know 'something' so long as we accept that something to be vague, personal and real only to us. It's fine to feel a little confused and lost. We all do from time to time. Then we surround ourselves with the familiar and trot on as best we can. That's okay too. However you choose to live and interpret the world I would recommend only this; be brave little soul. Put your faith in a greater scheme of something, if it suits you. If you choose simply to believe in life and happiness, rather than angels or abacuses, it is your belief and it will buoy you up on those days or weeks of uncertainty. Be as honest as you can, and treat everyone you meet as you would treat me, or your own child. Know that we are all innocents in our own ways, battling it out on the up and down landscape of life.

Your Dad has had an experience recently where he felt someone betrayed him and lied to him. He was angry with that person. Maybe it's my pregnancy hormones, or my spiritual hippy ways, but I couldn't wholly understand that anger. We have all hurt people, as much as they hurt us. We have all told lies. We all deserve a second chance. We all do the best we can with the tools at our disposal, and sometimes in times of confusion, depression or heartache, the only tool we feel we have is a lie, to betray, to do something that ultimately hurts someone else. This doesn't make us bad people. Like I said life is very complicated.

Your Dad has since had some further communication with that person. That person has been honest, he has admitted why he lied. He lied because he was embarrassed to tell the truth. Your Dad, being the good guy that he is now views this situation differently. But his initial anger sparked a wave of hurt feelings that none of us needed. But in this little incident, your Dad has forgiven, and the offending party has moved on a step. Second chances, my little darling, are essential.

When you look at the world as a mixed up and crazy place, and put yourself in other people's shoes, anger becomes a useless tool. Whilst I am sure you will feel anger and frustration throughout your life, I hope it only sparks through you briefly and is then dampened by the realization that all things are difficult, and making enemies of others is of no use. I hope no one hurts you. But this is life, and they will, as you will them. Inevitably. I know you though, and I know that in your soul, as in all our souls, you are good; you mean well, you have infinite love.

Hey little Poppyseed, dig deep into that love. Feel it, express it and give people a chance, at the end of the day, none of us know very much, not even the Einstein's among us... We are here for a fleeting few moments and the best thing is to embrace our unknowing and live within it, always with an eye to learning whilst recognizing that everyone we meet, from pauper to prince, are in the same boat. There is no room for hate in similarity, and trust me; we are all the same underneath.

Wishing you a lifetime of peace and understanding, Your Momma, Alice x

2 October 2012

Today was our first midwife visit, and last for a while too. Unless something goes wrong we are left to our own devices until later in the pregnancy. The midwife, Jo, was lovely, just how you imagine midwives to be. There was a lot of paperwork to fill out, lots of questions to try to figure out how much support we needed and whether or not we intended to do silly things such as smoke, drink, shoot heroin. I guess lots of people do…

There were also decisions to be made. Did I want the test for Downs Syndrome? This is a fairly innocuous question; lots of people have the test, as they want to know. But to me it was a loaded question. To me I was being asked, did I want to know, and if I did, and my baby had Downs Syndrome… what would I do about it? I hated it, I hated this question. It made me tear up and cry a little. I am in love with my baby already. I accept that child for what it is, what it has, who it will become. So no, I don't want the damned test. I'll take what I'm given and be happy with it. This child is indispensable, irrespective of disease, disability, drama, missing toes, whatever!

I didn't expect to have such a strong reaction. I really didn't. But at least I know where baby and I stand!

On a lighter note, James really does think he is a comedian. He has a standard joke he keeps rolling out whenever we are asked if we have any questions... He first unfurled the joke on the doctor at our appointment a week or so ago, and he of course let it out again for Jo's benefit. I have a feeling he may continue to use this…maybe forever. It's a little ridiculous, but yeah, it gets a giggle (and an eye roll) from me every time. So when Jo asked if we had any questions, James piped up with, 'Where do babies come from?' Oh god, he's only going to get worse…I can see it now on birthing day, him having a field day with all the doctors and nurses! Then to the teachers when baby starts school…then again on baby's graduation, wedding day, when baby has their own baby! It's never going to get old for him…I best steel myself for that! Or perhaps I ought to buy him a biology book and be done with it!

3 October 2011

Oh God I'm having a moment. I'm feeling emotional, and weird. I know it's nonsensical, and everything I am about to say is totally pathetic and whiney. But I'm going to say it anyway.

I feel like I'm all by myself. In fairness to my friends and family, I only really spent yesterday by myself, and even then I spoke to my Brother in Tokyo for forty-five minutes via the Internet. But still. I feel alone. Other people didn't answer their phones or didn't call me back. James is busy upstairs doing house renovations and I've been fine until maybe half an hour ago, but suddenly, the sun has set and I'm having a moment. I know I'm not lonely, but right now I feel that I am.

To counter this loneliness I thought about going to the gym to walk on a running machine. This I decided would make me feel weirder… Seeing all those old familiar faces who are there every day, but not actually speaking to anyone and certainly not telling them I'm pregnant. That is perhaps not a way to cure loneliness. Which leaves me with only one option I can think of; food shopping. All I feel I do right now is eat and sleep, so at least I'm feeding my habit. But that said, all I do is eat and sleep right now… I'm scared I will blow up like a whale, never lose the weight and be miserable forever. I must buy fruit, I must buy fruit. I must buy fruit.

Goddess, I'm being shallow and moaning, please help me.

I shall continue this self-sorry rant… What makes all of this worse is that I read an article about a footballers wife on her third pregnancy. A photo showed her at allegedly seven months pregnant, and the article discussed how she goes to the gym all the time. I haven't gone to the gym. I've done two pregnancy DVD's in as many days, and they were easy. I feel like a failure. Plus if she is that skinny at seven months I'm screwed. Realistically, I know the photo was probably fed by her marketing team, and was likely taken two months ago, but…she makes me feel bad about myself. I know better than this. I should not let this bother me. I should go meditate, but instead I'm going to go buy bananas – they have happy minerals in them, right?

Ok so I had a cry about all of the above. I know how stupid it is. I know I should be grateful, I know I should be counting my blessings, but there is something in those pregnancy hormones that renders the minutest things unbearable. I think I'll be ok, I'm composed and calm again. I'm going to take a deep breath and I'm going to do some food shopping…

...Apologies diary for my ranting, but it must be shared. I must be honest. There is no such thing as pregnant and perfect, as there is no such thing as soulfully complete. I guess I'll keep trying. And please be reminded that those spiritually calm souls such as Jesus, the Dalai Lama or Deepak Chopra have never had this hormonal junk to deal with – they are men. The bastards. I'm going to buy bananas. Wish me luck.

...Ok I'm back. As ever with my life I was gifted a little insight, one that put things back into perspective and helped me to find the gratefulness that I was desperately missing an hour or so ago. Wandering around the supermarket I happened across a couple with a young child in a buggy. They were bickering; or rather she was bickering with him. A stream of constant put downs fell out of her mouth, it was clear, to me a stranger, that she did not believe her partner to be good enough. He remained silent, and just let her go on and on. Their child, old enough to understand, was silent in his pushchair.

The energy that came from this couple really affected me. Whilst I'm sure the woman, in her own way, loves the man, her words and body language spoke very differently. It occurred to me that they were in a horrible rut, that the stress and strain of family life had torn apart what must at one point have been a happy union. Whilst I can't say this will never happen to me, between baby blues and life's hiccups, I could easily be her. But I will decide right now that this will not be me. All my moans and groans of before, are nothing. They are not real. I intend to move forward holding the things I love very close to my chest.

Thank goddess for bananas!

I have one final thing to note for today. I seem to be suffering from a form of evening time mental blandness. It gets to a certain time at night and my mind finds everything dull, dull, and dull. Television, film, radio, books, comedy, conversation, it's all just a boring shade of beige to me. The only answer I can seem to find for this is to go to sleep. Maybe it's a pregnancy form of tiredness, my brain is drained and it is done with anything stimulating, so refuses to join in with the outside world.

I wouldn't say this was frustrating so much. When it happens I'm too bored and bland to be frustrated. I'm feeling far too mundane to experience anything else. This evening I am going to try and spin it out for a while. I'll probably go to bed with a book, something salacious or gripping and see if that keeps me in any way alert. Though I know how this goes, I read one page and decide to rest my eyes. Before I know it I'm onto tomorrow. I hope this is a passing phase. That said, it's late, I don't care, whatever, talk to the hand, too bored for words. Yawn!

11 October 2011

Things have been better since my last entry, not quite so emotionally exhausting. The boredom has passed, and I have found myself staying up later, with more energy and interest. That said I don't feel wholly myself either. There is still occasional, and often lingering, nausea. Sunday saw me get up, eat breakfast and go back to bed simply because I could not be bothered to be awake through a nasty bout of sickness. But other than this, and the extreme tiredness that crops up randomly, I'm feeling great. Throughout this time I have been doing a lot of thinking about the recent past. I have been working things though my mind, considering them, looking at how far James and I have come…

The end of last year saw James and I hit a real stumbling block in our relationship, and our lives. He had been working probably twenty hours a day on releasing a single into the big, bad world. Being a perfectionist, he couldn't get to a place where he was happy with what he was producing, but a clock was ticking, promotion was happening. After years doing music in a number of bands, this single release suddenly felt like a make or break situation for him. The pressure was on, big time. Big, big, big time.

The lack of sleep, lack of anything other than pure stress over this damned song, caused all hell to break loose and our love took a direct hit. The lead up to this was a few months, maybe years, maybe a lifetime in the making. It coincided with being screwed over by a thieving manager, and a whole other host of negative outside influences determined to get their hooks into people they perceive to be successful in the music industry. It was messy.

To the outside world, what James was achieving was fantastic. But from my seat on the inside, all I could see was turmoil, inner agony and depression. I can't speak for him but what occurred next I can only describe as a breakdown, and I was there for the implosion, explosion, haunted house that followed, and the ride that eventually brought us to where we are now; back to life.

James's ride was my ride too. I truly believe that when something catastrophic happens, even if it is not directly stemming from your own issue, it is equally yours to deal with and it is down to you to examine yourself too. Whilst abandonment, separation, divorce or plain old nonchalance might protect from some more dire emotions, it is these emotions that are the calling card of something greater.

In James's agony, I was given a chance to not only dig deep and help him, but to also help myself. This was not an easy route to take. Watching someone have a breakdown, and witnessing their character change drastically, and for the worse, does not create a desire to 'make things work'. But at the same time the heart has a song that it must follow, sometimes even in spite of evidence that declares that song now null and void. The song of my intuition kept on pulsing despite advice and logic to the contrary. In following that song, and in re-finding both James, and myself, an unimaginable happiness has arisen. It was a hard slog. But it brought us here.

James has spent the best part of this year getting to grips with himself again, so have I. It's been a steep learning curve, we could have split, but I truly believe that after ten years together we weathered the storm and came out stronger. Whilst it was possibly the most painful thing I have ever lived through, I would not change it.

After ten years of being together, particularly through one's twenties, a lot of changes occur. We went from twenty-two-year-old party animals, to people with commitments, mortgages, him pursuing a music career, me pursuing a writing one. In many respects, this could most definitely have gone another way. Maybe when you look at how opposite we are, it should have. But it is in the main, our alter egos that are opposite. I know that in real life, all goals and ambitions aside, we get on well, we sympathize over the same things, we make each other laugh, and now we are becoming parents together. More than ever before in the last ten years, things finally feel right.

James and I have both chased and pursued our demons over the years. Being creative types has helped, and it has hindered. It was only since this 'make or break' set of circumstances that we focused less on our demons and more on ourselves, our true inner selves. You make a decision at some point in a loving relationship, to accept the relationship for what it actually is and what it could become, rather than reaching for the fantasy of Prince Charming or Miss Perfect. Neither really exists. All humans are flawed.

The sooner you realize that, and stop looking for freedom, redemption, happiness, success or perfection in another person's arms, the better. You can help each other find all of those things, but no way can a relationship in, and of itself, provide them. Fairytales and Disney have a lot to answer for in building up our hopes! Once the honeymoon has worn off, we all get dirt under our nails. James and I had some accepting to do, of ourselves and each other, and then some rediscovering. Rediscovering being the fun part, and is partially responsible for getting me pregnant!

Anyway I digress. The pressure of parenthood has been on. And whilst we have both made great inroads in 2011, James has felt a strong pull to take this further. A lifetime of a rock 'n' roll lifestyle (and trust me he started early) is a hard habit to break, but for the sake of everyone's sanity he has been doing that. And doing it well. My therapy course is helping me get to re-know myself too. We are both addressing our past selves and coming up smelling ever so slightly rosier.

It's an adventure of self-knowing and one that is bringing us tighter and closer. I love it, and I'm strangely grateful for all the horrendous crap that got us here. Crap really can turn out to be the most remarkable and transformative glue. We rode our darkest day and overcame it. In our divorce and dump society we did ourselves proud. I know we are going to be just fine. James is a man to be proud of, and I know a Dad to be proud of too in the not too distant future.

I know that the chaos we experienced occurred to bring in peace and make way for the light. Even in the bowels of our misery, I knew deep down that the pain we felt was right, was needed, and was what would take us forward. We swept our house clean, the cleansing process was exhausting and scary, but the end result is a fresh slate, and new beginning.

Our new beginning is happening together, and since the roller coaster stopped and we got off, I feel a sense of contentment and gratefulness that has never touched me before, because I never before had to fight so hard against the odds. The improvements in our lives have continued into this pregnancy, indeed pregnancy has given them more urgency and meaning. Now we go from making ourselves happy to preparation to make someone else happy.

This particular someone else is coming to us full throttle and with total innocence, as such the level by which happiness, calm and a 'happy home' is measured is demonstrably higher than it was when there was just the two of us. What was acceptable before, has now been automatically renegotiated. James and I have more work to do. But every step is a step closer to something stunning. Indeed, as we traverse our deep inner selves and transform our lives I suddenly have no time for nausea. Life is changing swiftly, love is changing with it, but I know that this is all for the best.

If I ever thought pregnancy and babies was all about measuring physical progress by weeks, and buying a decent pair of maternity jeans then I was wrong. Pregnancy is holistic and I am happy to say that that includes the whole unit, Momma, Poppa, Poppyseed, even the cats and rabbits will get a look in some way down the road as we change up their habits to make way for a little one. The home of course too is part of all of that. And great shifts have been happening in our space. Lots of jobs to be finished, rooms to be sorted, boxes to be moved, and later on, things to be made baby safe. It's a whole new world and James and I are like astronauts in training. Exploring inner space and reflecting the best of it outward into our lives.

Dear Poppyseed,
I dreamt about you last night. You were the most perfect little baby girl. You learned to crawl in one day and you pooped on my friends' carpet. I didn't know how to change your nappy, or how to breastfeed, but it didn't matter. You were stunning. The most amazing thing I have ever seen. I woke up very much in love with you. That feeling has not ebbed. You, my darling, are simply the best, and everything from now onward has you sat in the centre.

Mommy Alice xx

21st October 2011

It's been a while since my last entry. Let's put it this way, I haven't felt like writing. Every day has had it's own set of issues, but put into a concise list I have suffered the following in no particular order, constipation, trapped wind, bloating, exhaustion, nausea, headaches and above all... More bloating. I have had to become so conscious about what I put into my body, because when I get it wrong...oh how I have suffered. Bread has had to go, large meals have had to go, fruit and vegetables has taken over and finally things are calming down significantly. But a week of many varying distraught belly symptoms has been tiresome.

Because of all the bloating, I've noticed the miracle of the pregnant belly play out every single day. Each morning I wake up feeling my nice and slim self, by the end of day I have inexplicably bloated up to look and feel about six months pregnant. After a night of frequent toilet trips, and sleep driven expulsion of air (passing wind), each morning I am returned back to my fairly flat stomached self. And then as the day passes my stomach appears to advance several months in pregnancy again. This has been a source of confusion to many people. One night they will remark how I am suddenly showing, but by morning, that's all gone and no one can see a damned thing. Whilst this might be mildly amusing to read about, it's unpleasant.

Happily it's getting better, hence my renewed ability to write! I hope it stays this way. I also hope the bloat turns into a baby bump quickly as that would make the speculation so much easier to deal with.

Today I am pleased to report that I feel great. No nausea, no bloating and it seems that my conscious eating is paying off. Please goddess let it be paying off. I feel entirely normal today, other than frequent trips to the toilet to wee, I'm on top of the world. So much so, that I will be visiting the gym this morning.

The gym, now there is another subject. So many people have struck me down with a fear of the gym. A fear I thought was healthy. And yet whilst healthily afraid of the gym, I have been unhealthily bloated, horribly afraid of loss of body control, and feeling weaker, and weaker.

I have been advised now by many sources in the know, that exercise is brilliant in pregnancy. Of course I may not wish to jump around in the classes I enjoyed before pregnancy, I must be careful about getting too hot, or letting my heart beat go up too high. But this is all manageable. What matters most is keeping a decent level of fitness. The last thing I need is to sit on my bottom for the next seven months and suddenly find that I don't have the energy to keep up with a demanding newborn!

As the recent past has been a very physical time for me, there has been little space for the cerebral or the spiritual. I've been caught up in my body, though I hope that is ebbing away now. I'm looking after myself so well, and as a result any physical craziness is fading and setting me free to be me again. Being back at the gym is so right for me, eating well is so right for me, early nights are so right for me. All these things combined are creating happier times. I will listen to my body, I'll be a slave to my body, and I'll enjoy my body. And on that note…I need a wee. Chat soon…

…Wee over and now onto another subject….

Today I have been disgusted by the horror in the world. We are essentially living in barbaric times and I am happily bringing a sweet little life into all that. The news today has shown me at least two people, guilty of killing other people, trying to squirm their way out of it by manipulating the law, and another situation with the brutalized corpse of a much detested world leader being splashed all over the front pages of our Western Newspapers. Let's be honest the world can be a horrid place.

As a child I was scared of strangers, earthquakes, fires, of my parents dying, of animals becoming extinct, floods, wars and having no money. These childhood fears seemed very frightening and strangely likely, especially during the nighttime. Some of them were silly fears (such as Tsunami's when I lived in middle England) and were realistically nothing to get upset about. But the influence of mass media and news reports of such things happening in distant corners of the globe did not suffice to quell my childhood hysteria.

The scariest thing about the list of my childhood fears is that it's by no means exhaustive. Indeed, things to be afraid of have increased exponentially since the time that I was a child. And of course there is all the stuff that children don't know about, and that parents would rather they never knew about. I guess it suffices to let our children be aware only of their potentially unrealistic kiddy fears (such as a volcano hitting downtown Bolton).

No sane parent would make a child's fears worse by telling them the full extent of grotesque human behavior, potential catastrophe or indeed the other perils of planet earth that might befall anyone of us at any time. I'd reel off a list, but frankly, I don't want to depress myself!

Planet Earth is a beautiful and cruel place, as are it's master inhabitants; humans. It is intimidating to know I'll be setting a little soul loose on this place. It is no funfair. But what is a potential parent to do or think about any of this?

This is where I have to put my spiritual head on. I was once an innocent baby, and I came to this place, thus far I'm doing fine. People I know have suffered some horrific lifetime events, they too are doing fine. Essentially this life may not be a fun fair, but it is a playground of sorts. A playground that I believe we come to with purpose.

I don't believe souls are randomly developed here through biological processes. I believe souls are a part of this universe, a conscious part, a part that chooses to come here into a biological body. So whilst my little vulnerable baby will be in part sweet, innocent and in need of significant care s/he will also house a powerful soul. A soul that wishes to learn. A soul that came into this life with purpose, and for a reason. And part of that purpose will (I hate to admit it) include some suffering.

Yes, this life is horribly cruel, but it has its flip side. I also know that an acorn falls and spawns new life, and that everything here is a miracle. I know that some really cute animals exist; I know people can be incredibly kind. I know that love is more powerful than a nuclear weapon.

The world can be a scary place. Yet I believe that all things happen for a reason, karma is a great teacher and maybe right now I shouldn't focus on the world of the sensational. I will focus instead on my little world. The world that exists within the places I go, the people I see and the world of what is going on inside me. For me these things are all real. And whilst I know the world at large is busy obliterating itself, being nasty and getting it's hands grubby, I will focus on what I can control. I will focus on my moment. Let the world do what it will. I will practice and teach love and that is that. Maybe, just maybe, for my little kiddy I can make the world a funfair!

October 23 2011.
Well I have been through the full-on ups and downs of early pregnancy this weekend. Trying to maintain a sense of healthy, soulful values is darned hard work when on a beautiful, sunny Saturday morning, with not a care in the world, I couldn't stop crying! Yesterday I was an emotional wreck. Today I am perfectly content. Behold the joys of pregnancy.

I awoke Saturday after a lovely long lie in and I started to worry. I was worrying in particular that James and I were going out that evening. Instead of looking forward to an evening dressed up and watching live music with lovely friends, I became convinced of imminent disaster. I felt absolutely terrified about the prospect of the evening ahead and when James came in from doing Saturday overtime, I welcomed him with an offloading of my fears, which was soon followed up by floods of tears.

It makes no sense now. As a spiritual author who believes in what she warbles on about I know that there is no point or purpose in getting worried about something that hasn't even happened. But I spent the whole day getting myself in a heightened state of emotion about all the horrid things that could occur... Even as it came to getting dressed to go out, I sat on the bed and sobbed. I asked James if my boring, pregnant self was going to be a burden to his night out, he was sweet and told me in the nicest possible sense to get myself together, of course I wasn't.

Despite my hysterical reservations, it turns out my psychic sense was not correct in attuning to imminent disaster, but rather I was far off the mark. Far, far off the mark. We had a lovely night. It was a totally harmless, fun, pleasant evening with lots of lovely people and some fabulous music.

Now I am a big believer in intuition, but some wires got crossed with some mega hormones and my mental synapses responded all wrong to this circumstance, and that I guess is one of the curses of pregnancy. If you had asked me at noon yesterday what the night would hold, I would have told you my intuition was screaming doom and despair. But indeed doom and despair was not forthcoming. All was well.

Today I am feeling very much back to normal, and in retrospect, I can see that I was a hormonal crazy face. But what to do next time these fears hit, presuming, of course that they do? Well hopefully next time I may not take them so seriously. Really I could do with a litmus test for my hormones. Something I could dip into my ear and do a brief mental health check, because frankly my mental health was not great yesterday. And whilst this was a brief foray into the world of extreme unmindful thinking, it was not a pleasant one. I must now bear in mind, that what goes on in my mind, may not really be my mind, but may well be my little Poppyseed's developments causing my mind to temporarily lose itself. Happily, Poppyseed is worth it.

Now, on the same subject of pregnancy hormones, I have to wonder if I'm giving 'something off' to men in the near vicinity. I'm rarely, if ever approached by guys, and yet last night, all the drunkest and most offensive ones seemed to handpick me for their attentions. Perhaps their drunken minds recognized my relatively unstable one, saw a kindred spirit and took their chances… Alternatively, maybe I have started to 'glow', as a pregnant woman should. I may well be exuding some form of scent.

Who knows the cause of my sudden irresistibility? It is only unfortunate that the guys who did choose to flock to my side were frighteningly not my type and quite clearly under the influence of something other than just a few beers. Whilst I had a good night in general, these intimidating attempts at mating may well stand as solid reason why I should not leave the house again during pregnancy. I now attract scary weirdoes. Great stuff.

After yesterday's emotional blip, I woke today feeling terribly normal. I'm vaguely noticing a pattern. One day fine, the next day some combination of emotion / nausea / exhaustion. Which if the pattern is correct means that I am due for an off day tomorrow. Let's hope not as I have a long drive and two talks to perform to avid audiences as part of promotion for my last book. God forbid the audience is filled with drug addled lotharios come to witness me have an emotional breakdown.

Other items of note today: James and I are just getting on so well. Probably the best we have in a long time, maybe ever? Little Poppyseed has bonded us already and I feel utterly relaxed around him, and he clearly feels more himself than he has done for a long time. Having a joint goal is good for our souls, which in itself creates a beautiful prospect. James and I have always gone our separate ways, meeting at the end of the day for dinner and a daily round up. We have never really had a project or so much as a hobby together, apart from socializing and sharing a home of course.

James and I have always been two souls joined through love yet very separate in life. We were married, we had a house, we had cats, we chose to be together, but there was no weight, no gravitas, nothing other than some kind of mystery ingredient that draws people together and makes them stay together through thick and thin. But ten years down the line the idea of having a little babe together has drawn something in us closer, I guess it's the F word – family. I love that F word.

October 29th 2011

What a fabulous week. Not because of any great life-changing miracle, but simply because I have felt almost normal. Every night I have been up beyond my previous pregnancy bedtime, and I've been a busy girl. On Monday I gave two talks in Bristol, Tuesday I did my usual meditation teaching in the evening, Wednesday I went to a crazy rock gig, Thursday I saw my best friend Roisin and then Friday I made a homemade pie from scratch, pastry and all! Tonight I'm off to some little village for a swish and fancy style music event. All I can say is, thank goodness the hormones have relaxed on me this week or else I may well have gone into hiding.

Other than the occasional bout of deeply painful stinging nipples, all has been well. This nipple thing is actually worth more of a mention. I keep having attacks of what feels like someone is lighting my nipples on fire. It's bearable, but only just. It lasts around ten minutes and it makes me want to sob. Then it vanishes as quickly as it arrived. Thankfully it isn't occurring too often. I guess the boobages are getting ready for the babe.

Feeling in good health (other than the nipple attacks) has been of great assistance in getting to have some time to think about life. It sometimes has felt I've been so consumed in how I'm feeling in my body that I forget to go beyond the physical or emotional to examine my soul. So in-between events this week I have taken time out to meditate with my belly out, hands on top, connecting with the little soul inside.

I am not the only one wishing to connect with the little soul in my tummy. A few people have taken to speaking to me with their hands on my belly, or when greeting me with a hug, their hand goes to my tummy. This is unnerving. I have always had a hang up about my stomach. It's the first area to gain weight for me, and if I have a very human 'down' moment, it is usually belly related. So to suddenly have people stroking, holding and gazing at my vaguely rounded tummy is really most unnerving.

I can't help but consider that all they are doing is cradling my fat. It's too early surely for them to connect with anything other than my spare tyre? Possibly they may encounter rumblings of a belly too full of bread and having a bad reaction? But if it makes them happy…who am I to turn tummy Diva? Imagine that, little old spiritual me throwing up a hissy fit because some poor well-meaning friend decided to pet my bump. No, I think I'll have to get used to the belly gazers. Which, as belly gets bigger, and I become more certain they are petting baby rather than bloat, I will no doubt become happier about.

Now, they say that pregnancy brings on an upturn in the world of the senses, particularly smell, and of course taste, as we allegedly hanker after anything from jellied eels through to coal. But what about the spiritual sense, the psychic sense and the intuitive sense? Well, this week I have had a few things happen that were simple, nothing profound, but otherwise unexplained.

It started Monday when James got up to go to work and I was

laid in bed snoozing. I was having random thoughts about a big, beautiful white cat that had visited us a few times last year. I never saw the cat again and I was vaguely pondering on how much I wished it would come back – I had it ear marked as a new member of my animal family. Anyway, before James left, he was waiting to be picked up by his lift to work. He shut his eyes for a quick doze and apparently sensed something staring at him in the living room. He opened his eyes to see the very same white cat staring at him. He chased it out (bah humbug) and then shouted up to me that the white cat from last year had been in our house! How very awesome. Some part of me connected with the big white dude, and whilst I'm sad husband did not welcome him with open arms, I hope that our apparent psychic connection will let Mr Cat know he is welcome back anytime.

Later that same day, I was driving over to my Mum's when I entertained a passing fancy in my mind that when I arrived they would give me some chocolate tiffin cake. Not chocolate fridge cake as they have so often given me before, but actual gooey, crunchy stunning yummy Tiffin. On arrival the first thing Karen, my Mum's partner, said to me was, there is some Tiffin in the kitchen for you. A whole pot of it cut into little chunks just for me. Well I've been told since, that it was actually for James too, but needless to say, barring one piece that I donated to my Mum, I scoffed the lot! Delicious.

So my psychic senses appear to have amped up, although not about anything vastly important or life changing. This spiritual heightening is just the kind of thing I had hoped and expected as part of the spiritual journey that this pregnancy is for me. Indeed in Bristol this week I had a tarot card reading, and it turns out that the pregnancy, much as I am expecting, will help me find my place in the world, as a mother, as an author, as a person. Indeed that's the second reading I have had where that has been said, and it rings true because I sense it myself. I feel it in my overactive waters! I am feeling more whole as a person than I ever have before. My perspective is so much clearer and I am happy in my flesh knowing that from my flesh something so precious will come.

Having a child is helping me to surrender and release so much junk. All of those negative thoughts, the 'what ifs', they all drop away. It's just me and thee, Poppyseed, and Dad too of course, and the cats, and the rabbits… but yeah you get what I'm saying. Life is looking very different. I feel safe, protected, wise almost. The whole world looks nicer and people in general all have a glimmer, because at the end of the day, they are all someone's son or daughter. We are here to give life, and what goes on beside that with our careers, our reputations, our possessions, they are all distractions. What matters are our relationships; including the ones you grow yourself from seed! As well as the ones you find in the fields of life and fertilize with fancy dinners cinema trips and gossip.

It's been an intriguing week and whilst I am succumbed to my internal eventualities, Mr James has been busy tearing bits of the house down. It's been dusty to say the least. James has been so hard working, but of course it is all worth it. We have roughly six months to create something special, a nicer place to live, a good parenting station. Alongside this we have a relationship to polish off and get as right as is humanly possible. I am confident we are right on track. And other than the occasional niggling (from me – I admit it I am a grump at times) we are so very happy still. Happy maybe isn't even the right word; happy has a birthday style hysterical edge to it. We are content. We are really, brilliantly content. I now need to go get ready for a fancy night out, and in-between make up application and clothing choices I must remember to place my hands on my belly and breathe.

October 30th 2011
A few thoughts on exercise... I believe that if you feel able, then exercise is very important in pregnancy. Whilst I am growing a new person, I too am still a person; a person who loves working out, it keeps me sane. I've chosen to ignore all the naysayers who panic if I mention doing exercise and trust that my body knows what it wants and needs. And what it needs, on occasion, is exercise. I'm clearly not going to start training for a marathon, but keeping up trips to the gym is essential for my wellbeing. I do this with full consideration to my baby's wellbeing of course.

Having spoken to a number of personal trainers, the consensus is that exercise in pregnancy is not to lose weight, or build muscle, but to keep fit, to keep on top of what you already have. I am further informed to be sure not to allow my heart rate go over 140. For a lady who normally hits 170 BPM's, this active attempt to go slower is hard work. I feel like my gym session has become all about not sweating, not panting and not feeling the burn. I miss the burn, I miss the breathlessness, and I miss the sweat. That said, as long as I'm moving and keeping mobile, I can make up the sweat loss during the occasional hot flush!

To my mind, exercise is a spiritual necessity. We are here in a physical form, and that form needs to move, it needs to groove, it needs to be honed in whatever way suits. That may be yoga, gym sessions, walking, gardening or swimming. It doesn't really matter, but what would matter is spending my whole pregnancy on the couch only to find that I couldn't change a nappy without getting breathless, or that when it comes to chasing a crazy toddler about, I can't keep up as my muscles have atrophied.

In pregnancy, we have a nightmare host of hormones throwing themselves our way, and exercise, no matter how soft and easy, is of assistance to the body. It raises your endorphins and when faced with nausea or grumpy moments then I need all the endorphins I can get! I do not see pregnancy as an excuse to allow everything to be done for me. I intend to keep carrying my own shopping bags and opening my own doors until such time as belly no longer allows it. I am pregnant, not disabled, and I will take pride in doing what I did before. Unless a Dr orders otherwise, then nothing (much) changes.

My other thought for the day is all about Hypnobirthing. I just ordered a book and downloaded a free application. Both on the subject of positive, natural, drug free birthing through hypnotherapy. It seems that hypnobirthing is all about removing the fear and allowing birth to be as easy, natural and calm as is possible. So I guess this is my birth plan…that and a water birth at a birthing centre – no doctors or medications allowed. More on this later, I'm still getting my head around it. All I know is that I want the birth to be a natural affair, as much as I can possibly control that… If I am destined to have a caesarean due to complications, then so be it, all things happen for a reason. But if the choice is mine, the hypno/water magic is the way forward. I think I may have found something quite wonderful in hypnobirthing, a viable, incredible alternative to screaming my way through birth and demanding an epidural. I guess I'll keep you posted.

31 October 2011

Happy Halloween! Or indeed Samhain, as I'm feeling more Paganly inspired. Samhain existed long before the familiar traditions of modern Halloween. Samhain really marks the end of summer, and has come to be linked with other traditions that involve the veil between the other side and earth being thinnest, and therefore the ghosts and the ghouls

This Samhain is pertinent for me because the end of summer really marks the end of my singledom in the world. Of course I am in a relationship, but when I say single, I mean my only-ness, my me-ness, the end of Alice the woman who can do what she wants, and the beginning of Alice, the woman with serious commitments, Alice the woman who has spawned a whole new person.

Whilst I may have possessed a reasonable level of maturity before, I am now becoming an official grown up. You could say that the summer of my life is behind me, and the mature, cogent, real colors of autumn are upon me, a little older, a little wiser, and a little less free. It's time to drop my leaves and give back. Return my nutrients to the soil and allow them to bloom next year in the new generation that I am carrying. I like the idea of dropping my leaves, stripping back; giving so much of myself to someone whose life is in gestation, yet to start. Let my child have all my leaves. It is Poppyseed's time. I will instead grow wrinkles and try to dispense wisdom. But the leaves, the flush green leaves of youth, and the blossom that comes with it, they are for my baby now. I can totally live with their loss, happily.

I didn't start the day off feeling so philosophical. This morning I was visited by a serious case of the extreme grumps. I would even go so far as to say I felt angry. I felt angry and sick. I was being completely irrational, but I was, at the least, aware of how ridiculous I was being.

The most inane things were sparking my anger. A lovely, kind friend texted to ask how we were, and the first flush of fuming was upon me. I couldn't help but see it as nagging, digging, looking for fault. I tried to explain this to my friend Claire, who luckily was having none of my nonsense and told me so directly.

I realized quickly that this reaction was hormonally inclined and totally nonsensical. In that knowing, I found some sanity. In my sanity, I decided to listen to meditation music to try and chill myself down a notch or two. This infuriated me more, as I couldn't help but think it sounded excessively twinkley. But I persevered. I drank some water. I dealt with some nausea and an hour or two later I was more or less back to normal.

With my hormonal fit behind me, I have gone on to have some

interesting thoughts. A lovely friend of mine is also pregnant, a little ahead of me, and has been giving me some much-needed guidance. She suggested I check out attachment parenting. Having looked into this, it pretty much describes the way I want to raise my baba. Basically I want to love it up, let the little fella know he or she is much loved, and appreciated. I want to give them a big place in my world, and in turn the whole world. I want to be attached.

Now here comes the sticking point. According to much spiritual theory, and my own previous writings, attachment is bad. Attachment lends us to place our mental and spiritual wellbeing on things external to us. It is thought that this is not realistic because these are not things we can actually control, and we are better off looking to our inner selves. Now maybe this is just a matter of wording and semantics, but it's worth thinking about.

Attachment has its meanings. It's definitely bad to be attached to outcome, to possessions, to the material world. It's even bad for our emotional health to be overly attached to people, places, and pets. I try to set others free, and I want them to do well and live their lives, but I am attached to my husband, I am attached to my friends and family. I like them all very much indeed. If they died that attachment would be extremely evidenced by my broken heart.

But maybe here I am not talking about attachment but love. I love my friends, James, my family. I love my unborn baby. Essentially I can control very little. I cannot control what any of these people do. But I can love them, from a place of genuineness. So this is how I will choose to view 'attachment' parenting, as simple, plain, old-fashioned loving parenting. And if you love someone you set them free, and hope that some form of bond has been created that means they will come back as and when the time is right. The same rings true for kids. Not to say I plan to dump my five year old in a park and see if s/he returns, but rather that I will love my child dearly, and guide them to the best of my abilities. Yet simultaneously I will make a conscious decision to let them be who they are, and continue to love them no matter what.

Healthy attachment is love and caring by another word. Unhealthy attachment is obsession and over reliance. And whilst I will happily surrender the negative aspects of attachment, I am not prepared to release the love, the passion, and the natural motherly concern. I am sure that at times the lines between good attachment and bad attachment will be blurred. When my little one brings home Mr or Miss Inappropriate, or commits their first misdemeanor, or throws an earsplitting tantrum. At times like this I am convinced that the good / bad lines of attachment will get confused. But that is life right? We all get it wrong occasionally, baby and me. Aiming for perfection is all very well and good, but like my child will mess up a million times, as will I.

Attachment should be taken with a pinch of salt, replaced with a dollop of love and a consciousness that keeps us aware not of fear or worry, but of love and guidance. Big words for a woman who is still in her first trimester. I know this. But we must think beyond our morning sickness some days. Life is being grown; the least I can do is plan how I intend to embrace that life. With a little healthy, happy attachment and a whole universe of love.

✡

Dear Poppyseed,
Today is 2nd November 2011, and on this day, ten years ago, your Mum and Dad first met. We have been together a whole decade, quite an achievement I feel. The best thing is, that whilst we have loved each other, and been friends all this time, it is really your existence in our world that has brought us closer. Knowing you

are on your way has forced us out of bad habits, and into a place where we are prepared to live life very differently. Your existence, at only eleven weeks old, has done the work of a hundred therapists. You have solidified us as a happy, loving couple.

Particularly, you have helped your Dad like you would not believe. A few days before I realized I was pregnant with you, I was discussing the possibility of pregnancy with Dad. I was having odd bad ache, and I suspected strongly that I was 'with child'. As the conversation ended, your Dad chipped in, almost under his breath, 'I hope you are pregnant'. Which to many happy couples may seem like the norm, but for us it meant so much more.

Your Dad has been a bit of a Peter Pan over the years, refusing to drop bad habits, living a crazy lifestyle as though he is indestructible. He has struggled with a few addictions that have, at times, threatened to tear us apart. He has struggled to be himself. When he said that he hoped I was pregnant, he realized that a third party, one who comes in and blasts new air, was what he needed, the incentive he desired to get himself on the straight and narrow.

And as I sit here, ten years into our relationship, I can see a litany of happy times and hard times scattering our past. It's only in the past few months that we have truly come together to overcome this past barrage of chaos. Whilst there was a reason we stayed together ten years, it is only now I can really feel it. Maybe we should have invited you into our lives earlier!

At least Dad and I can both say we have done an awful lot of things. Your Dad has created amazing music, for several years, even releasing a single and featuring in newspapers and magazines. I've written my books, which were published and had nice little things shoot off from that. We are both still in our day jobs, and have not as yet set the world on fire. But that's cool. Life is as it is, and quite frankly I'd rather have you, than a bestselling book, or a rock star husband. If those things happened alongside you, then that would be wonderful. But if not, who cares! There is so much more to life than fulfilling ambitions.

Success can only truly be measured by happiness.

The happiness found in achievement, in the material world, is brief, delusional and full of empty sagging lust. The happiness of loving relationships, of life, of everyday miracles is far more lasting, far more fulfilling. Do whatever you want in life my baby, but never forget who you are and the people that matter.

Anyway, you are far too young for such lectures! I guess instead I'll tell you the story of how your Mum and Dad met.

I was out partying one night with my friend Laura. Laura and I had met at a temporary job. We worked together one day, and I walked out of the job because the boss had returned from holiday, neglected to notice that I had revamped her entire filing system and instead gave me a talking to about being lazy. I had nothing to lose, having only just moved to Leicester, and cock sure of myself to get another job, I went on my lunch and never returned. In spite of our brief knowing of each other, Laura and I kept in touch (we still are friends) and became, for a little while, regular girls about the town together.

On one of these nights she and I ended up in a club called Weavers. We were mooching about on the dance floor when some longhaired dude walked past. Now, what do you do when this happens? Well in your Mum's twenty-two year old eyes, there was but one option. I pulled his hair. He turned round, came over and asked me 'do you know how f**king gorgeous you are?' To which I went all shy and giggly. He was quite the charmer, foul language aside. But he went his way and I went mine.

Not much later Laura and I decided to wander the rooms of the club, no doubt looking for totty; on my part the longhaired dude. We found him. He saw me, I saw him, eyes across the room and all that… I begged Laura not to leave me when I saw him headed my way. I had not been long out of a relationship and I wasn't so sure of myself. Of course Laura ignored me completely and disappeared into thin air. Leaving me sat like a nodding dog, unable to speak to this guy who was persevering beyond belief to have a conversation with me. That guy was your Dad, and persevere he did, because…well look what happened.

I don't remember much of our one-way conversation. He definitely told me he was in a band. I definitely was impressed. But I definitely did not show I was impressed. I probably played it cool; so cool I barely spoke. We certainly ended up smooching in the courtyard outside, and I remember some girl he knew coming over and saying how cute we looked together. He then remembers Laura and I leaving in a taxi with two random guys she had picked up and heading off home. As for the random guys, I don't know who they were and they jumped out of the taxi and ran off refusing to pay. Nice.

Your Dad and I had swapped numbers, and the next day my phone came everywhere with me. I believe that when he called I was in the shower. I stopped the water and played it cool...again. He asked if I wanted to go out that night. I said I didn't know and I'd call him back. Of course I wanted to…but instead I went and consulted with my neighbor Mark on this matter. Mark told me to go for it, so I texted back a time and place. Then Mark and I went to the local country park, got stoned and visited a pub where we sank a few strong cocktails. Classy pre-date preparation, I'm sure you'll agree! Mark was out with his friends that night at a place called the Orange Tree. So that was where I met James. He dragged a friend along too and it was all very awkward.

He didn't realize that I barely knew the people I was with, having only lived in Leicester for a month or so. So he went about trying to impress my friends. He still teases me today about the paint-splattered trainers I turned up in to that first date. My only excuse being was that I was fresh out of being a student, and paint splattered trainers were all the rage at

Lancaster University, I am sure.

As the night went on we sectioned ourselves off, to the point we decided to ditch the others. We walked several miles back to my house and then stayed up all night just talking. The next morning he nipped out to the shop, and just when I thought he may never return he came back with a cheap bunch of shop front flowers and a nice big bottle of vodka. Romance at it's height, might I add! In retrospect, I do not approve, but I was young. I hope when you are dating Poppyseed, that it is all museums, fine food, champagne and picnics in fields! We then carried on drinking and talking for the rest of the day. So rock 'n' roll, so different to how I am now. But the truth... In this beginning, a billion future problems with drink and late nights were seeded, but more than that, one great big fat true love story had commenced. We have lived through the late nights and partying, and yet the love remains, catalyzed now in the form that is you.

We have both changed so much. I did a lot of my changing a couple of years back. Your Dad got a bit delayed back in 2010, but he has done a sprint and is about ready to over take me any day now. He better get ready because in a month or two he is going to be not only my number one fella, but the one upon whom I totally rely. I love that. Me and Mr James; a crazy, zany, vodka fuelled love affair. Vodka is now well and truly behind us and in its place has come sanity, spirituality and next up a little Poppyseed will be born. The biggest adventure yet.

✡

November 9th 2011

I had a list of things I was going to write up in this diary. Yesterday it seemed radically important that I discuss with these pages the misery of my mood swings. Nausea, exhaustion, the fact chocolate makes me feel sick, negative thinking and general pathetic-ness. But as it happens I awoke today in a fabulous mood and it has continued to get better as the day has passed. So I won't bore you with the horrid details of my inner mind as affected by pregnancy hormones and a big dose of feeling sorry for myself. It happened, trust me, it wasn't pretty, but today the sun is shining so we will concentrate on that.

Instead, I will say only this. Life is hard. Things hurt us. But dwelling on them makes no difference. Dwelling on them, when in fact we have already surpassed, surmounted and conquered those things, is just plain daft. Put it this way. For the past few days 'plain daft' has been a pretty good description of me.

Then, last night, I did an accidental mediation. The TV wouldn't work. Or should I say I was having a dim moment, was totally tired and couldn't figure out how to work it. So I decided a few moments without distraction would be the best thing for me. I sat back on the sofa and I let the thoughts come. I was flooded over by the wonderfulness of my circumstances. Yes I had been through some awful stuff earlier this year, but it got me here, it got me pregnant, it got me happy. And with that accidental meditation my whole outlook on life turned around.

I picked up my happy self where I left off. I remembered the teachings of my last book, I remembered who I was, I remembered my smile and I forgot all about the bitching, moaning and whining of my hormone addled brain. Life is good. Life is far, far better than it ever was. Life is going to get even more superb with each passing day. I am doing really well. I must remember to remember that. Thank golly that the TV broke. Thank goddess that some unconscious wisdom or divine interventions shook me out of myself.

Anyway Alice is back in the room. She is currently making a vegetable curry, and she is smiling.

11 November 2012
Apart from constant trips to the loo and a tad bit of nausea, things are well. I made a trip to the gym today and walked on the running machine. Looking around I was surrounded by Women in lycra, women with fabulous figures. They were all huffing and puffing away, trying to craft their physicality's into something from their mind desires. I have to say that I thought they all looked tremendous. I wondered to myself, do they have any idea how good they look? The answer is that no, they probably don't. They are probably so focused on some problem area, as I always was, that they can't see the true picture.

The true picture is that they looked damned fine, toned, slim, some not so slim but still sexy, gorgeous. Pregnancy is not turning me lesbian, but these girls were hot. And I know they had little or no idea of this hotness. Maybe one day they too will be pregnant like me, surrounded by gorgeous women and they will have a realization that they were always far more perfect than they realized. Because that is what I realized today, I too, pre-pregnancy was fine and hot and all of that. But I couldn't see it. All I could see was tummy fat. What I didn't realize was that no one cared about my tummy fat. With or without it, I was fine as I was. Damn. Now I'm 'glowing' and on a good day still relatively unpregnant looking. But I feel this appreciation of my previous body has come too late, I wish I'd known it at the time.

Maybe this is why women who have had children tend to come across so confidently. Because they now appreciate what they have in terms of physical health, and the fact that their body can turn out miracles. Am I on the verge of a whole new way of body definition? I think perhaps I am. Once this little baby is born I have a feeling I am going to love myself in a whole new way. Saggy skin and potential stretch marks aside, my female form is a work of wonder. I'm never going to moan about my belly again.

Whilst I was contemplating all of this physical philosophy, I did a side-glance and saw my own reflection in the gym mirror. I look bloated – I'm not moaning! I wasn't sure if I looked pregnant or just like I had a bad period. I do look pregnant to me. But to others I may just look like I'm carrying excess weight on my belly. As such I am pregnant in disguise. I can hide amongst the gym's fit folk without disapproving looks or glances at my big round belly shifting about on the cardio equipment.

I do feel a little like I need to hide my exercising. I'm proud of doing it, and anyone who asks, I would happily tell them. But at the same time I know so many people disapprove. You simply do not see pregnant women in gyms. I saw one once, and I did in fact stare a little. I didn't disapprove, but I may have wondered about the ladies motivation. That was years ago though, and now I wouldn't have such thoughts. I'd no doubt think 'go on sister' get that blood pumping, burn off your frustrations, be healthy! Yet everyone has an opinion on a pregnant woman moving her ass too much. I refuse to succumb to anyone's cotton wool approach. So I sucked my tummy in – very good for posture during pregnancy - and I carried on walking at a reasonable pace, keeping my heart rate down but allowing my limbs to enjoy some oxygen.

13 November 2012

I hope my cats are going to be okay with the baby. I know that Jimi cat is so laid back he may barely notice. Molly cat however is an entirely different case. She has been my baby for the longest time. She is my shadow. She adores me, and I adore her. We are the best of friends even across the barrier of species. Her turf is seriously going to be encroached upon by this new arrival. I have explained it to her. I do tell her things in the hope that she may understand, or perhaps that her soul may understand. She has given little indication of understanding. I would say she is being more needy than ever, but she has always been needy towards me. Like I said, I'm her mum. I have been for six years.

I guess I'll keep reminding her of her approaching human sibling and I'll offer out a little more love. That, and at some point I must wean her out of sleeping in the bedroom next to my bed, because that is where baby will go. A direct replacement. She won't be happy. So the weaning may have to start soon so that Molly does not see the direct correlation of baby in, cat out. I'm determined to juggle this well. People tell me that the cats will not mean anything to me once the baby is here. I tell people they clearly do not know me. Love is love and I love them puddies.

Dear Poppyseed,
Today I have something I feel I need to share with you. You are your life. You have all the power in the world. Your life is as you believe it to be, as you dream it to be. You can create your own existence happy or otherwise, starting by living with an awareness of your thoughts. Everything is your choice; even those things and times when you feel you have no choice. You always have a choice, and whilst this choice may feel limited, it can define a lifetime for better or worse, depending upon how you choose to embrace it.

Joy and pain are all in your grasp. They too are your choice. Your mistakes are natural rites of passage, they are learning. You create you from the things you do wrong and the things you do right and how you choose to move through everyday. You own your self and your experience in this lifetime.

Remember this baby, when life lets you down and things seem awry, know that it is in your power and choice to see and feel things differently, to make your thoughts happier and in turn watch dirt turn to gold. You have a magic touch my Poppyseed; don't let anyone tell you different. Don't allow others to dictate your choices or limit your happiness. There are no limits and choice is ever present. Know this little baby and from this perspective you can change your world.

15 November 2011
We had our first baby scan today! What a magical, exhilarating and wonderful experience. The first glimpse of my little baby took my breath away; I so hoped the lady with the scanner would linger there all day. Of course that wasn't going to happen. But the five-minute glimpse we got of the little miss or mister was so perfect.

The side effect being that James and I are grinning like buffoons, hugging each other at every random opportunity and generally being a real pair of happy heads. We also had our first browse through some baby clothing catalogues; trying to figure what may suit the black and white bean baby we saw dancing on the scanner screen.

Having had two close friends recently lose their babies at the first scan we hadn't been taking anything for granted. We were nervous as we drove to the hospital and nervous as we waited. We have placed a huge amount of love and emotion on our little baby bean, and it is not beyond the realms of possibility for something to go wrong, it happens all the time, one in five I believe. Horrible odds.

James was eerily quiet as the magnitude of what might happen in that room dawned on us. I chirped away like a happy little bird, determined to think positive, determined to stick to what my deep inner self was telling me. And my deep inner self was well aware that all would be fine and dandy. In this instance, thank the cosmos, it absolutely was. Everything was wholly in order, baby is healthy and so mum and dad can breathe again. We are blessed and lucky that everything is fine and it is only with this knowledge that we can now start to look ahead thinking prams, nappies, romper suits and cots.

Now me being me, means something spiritual generally has to happen. And today, as well as the obvious, something else rather special happened too. As we were hanging around in the scanning reception (me complaining of needing the toilet due to the necessity for a full bladder) the scanning room door opened, and there stood a lovely friend of ours, Kim. She clearly hadn't told us she was pregnant, and we are now sworn to secrecy as her pregnancy has more complications than the norm. But whilst it wasn't a purposeful intrusion, I hope it was, in some respects, a pleasant one for her. Her husband works away so she was there alone. Even if our presence was a shock, at least she got to chat to some friendly faces. And of course I have found myself another Mommy-to-be friend! Ah how I love a happy coincidence.

As of today, the world at large now knows about our expectant bundle of joy as per our unavoidable facebook announcements. Today was very cool. I fell in love with a little squirming black and white image and James and I had a little renewal in our own right too. Babies are the best. Babies rule the World. Babies are the key to world peace. Goodnight.

16 November 2012

Several years ago someone was murdered and because of him a department was set up, rules implemented, staff employed and hope gifted out. Because of this murder I have a job. The job pays well, has benefits and has added significantly to my life. It has allowed me to buy a house, buy clothes, nice food and run a car. Because of this, I have had time to write books and do the things that I enjoy in this lifetime. It hasn't mattered if I make money from the books, because I have had a job, a job created as a result of that dark awful death. I have free time and spare time and I have enough spare cash to dine out, party, and buy things I don't always need. I live a nice life. I am by no means rich in finances, but I do okay, I cover my costs, I feel secure despite a recession.

And all of this is possible because several years ago, someone was murdered and instead of that murder going unsolved or unreported, it was a big, fat, massive deal. The world changed a little as a result. So did my life, although I did not see it at the time. Maybe I didn't really see it until today. Today I am grateful, I am humble and I resolve to be more appreciative of what I have been gifted as a result of this. We are all so connected. One storm can create a ripple elsewhere and vice versa. I have been on a ripple of benefit, from another family's horror, loss and tragedy. Because of that loss I can bring my child into the world and I can provide for that child nicely. What a horrendous beautiful ripple I have ridden. For that I can only be thankful.

17 November 2012

So far today I have taken scissors to my tights to create a little extra room. I have undone my top button, not to be sexy, but to allow blood to my bosom. I have also fixed my cardigan shut with a safety pin. Time to buy some maternity clothes I think…

This afternoon a lady I know fairly well asked me if finding out I was pregnant 'was a shock'. This may have just been a badly phrased question, but I found the implication to be a bit off. It suggests that the pregnancy was an accident, that I do not want the baby, and that perhaps the questioner thinks I'm not cut out to be a mum.

Was it a shock? Your question is a shock! Hell no lady, it was no shock!

Maybe I'm reading too much into this. I will let it go and put it down to a woefully worded query. Nothing more, nothing less. However, I can't help feeling irked by the question. I can't help thinking it reveals what that person really thinks of me. I should be a little more soulful about this, but this pregnancy is the best thing that ever happened to me, and the question just seems dirty. I won't dwell on it. I will take a deep breath and let it go.

I'll leave it at that. I could easily turn unspiritual and rant about this. But no, there was no shock here. Naught but love and joy. Love and Joy.

Let me change the subject… Have I mentioned the mind-numbingingly painful stingy nipples I keep getting? It can occur anytime, anyplace, and when it does, it literally feels like they are doused in acid. It makes me miserable. It's awful. Pressing them really hard seems to work, sort of... But in general, it's just pure pain. I can only hope it does not last the whole pregnancy.

…This evening I spoke online to a friend in a foreign country who is also pregnant. She is doing well with her pregnancy, though I think she is reticent to get too involved because she sadly lost a previous baby, quite recently and in the early stages. My heart goes out to her on that. Once you know you are pregnant you put a ridiculous amount of hope and heart into that little embryo. Too much perhaps… I know I did. As such, she is now a little unwilling to get excited or to believe things will be okay. But all is well, and I feel it will continue to be well for her. I feel so grateful too for my healthy pregnancy. One day our babies will play together, I know it.

18 November 2012

My day at work left me feeling most grateful of the relative smoothness of my own life. So many people live dangerous, dirty, destructive existences and that is just so regular and normal for them. Chaos and mayhem is the definition of their week. Whilst my life certainly has had its ups and downs I am hugely grateful that I am unlikely to ever descend into that kind of drama. I pray for those whose lives are infiltrated by such turmoil. I hope that they can find some peace, because seriously, there are some messed up situations out there, and some messed up people. Sometimes those of us on the right side of the tracks just don't know we are born.

I've been wondering today also about whether babies fix people. I know having a baby is no way to save a relationship, any agony aunt worth her salt will tell you that. But does bringing a new person into your life present an opportunity to pimp and perfect yourself? Well yes, of course it does. I suppose not everyone takes that opportunity. But it is an opportunity nonetheless.

James and I have been working on 'us' for a little while prior to being pregnant. I have mentioned that things had taken a bit of a nosedive and we were finding our way back. Having this baby together has been like a big road sign, giving us clear directions and at the same time taking us along a magical track whereby we rejuvenate and refresh our love in the wonders of everyday miracle. Having our baby and doing so consciously is a cure I never expected.

In having a child life-purpose is gifted with a big fat ribbon. Previous to this we both had individual purpose, he did music, I wrote. But the purpose of a child, the business of a child, this is some serious shizzle. This is hardcore purpose. This is undeniable, selfless, enlightening purpose. It is far more important than our hobbies/careers, no matter how successful those things may one day become...or not. This is purpose that requires us to step up, and out of our bubbles and make a real tangible difference, on a daily basis. This is so fucking real.

As humans we are designed biologically to mate and reproduce. But add a dose of love and respect to that and you are literally flying high. I am in bliss right now. My husband is a changing man. He is doing himself justice after years of scraping the barrel. This baby is showing him his potential, his ability, and his wondrousness. Neither of us are existing for what we might be one day and instead we are existing in what we are now. It's a change in perspective that alters everything for the better.

James's spark of inner amazingness has truly soared. It is like watching an awakening or enlightenment first hand. In turn I too am becoming better. We are both being kept on our toes. We are changing and with each change the other person is challenged in new and healthy ways. We have to keep up with one another, and we do so out of love, not necessity or desperation. This time of our lives, as we prepare to be parents is eye opening, transformative, hard work and utterly inspiring. At the heart of it all sits a Poppyseed.

19 November 2011

Went maternity bra shopping today and this turned out to be deeply distressing. There was not a single bra in the well-known store that fit me. Not a one. They were all too small. I don't consider myself a large person; I'm a UK size twelve, or ten on a blue moon. Yes, my boobs are on the big side at the best of times, and pregnancy has seen them swell. Yet I can't believe it should be so traumatic to get a bra. If me, with my fairly average body shape, is struggling, lord knows how bigger people cope, or indeed smaller people who remain tiny but with a swelling bust. Not good enough world…we need more bras, in more sizes, in better colors, with matching knickers. Am I really asking too much?

Needless to say I didn't purchase a booby sling. Instead I got tearful, resolved to continue strapping up in a sports bra and went home miserable.

21 November 2011
Being spiritual really doesn't matter. It's living that does. Having a soulful heart is key to all things. But 'spirituality' as a tool, a key, a defense, a skill is not essential.

People live beautifully, everyday without an ounce of faith. What counts, and hell let's be clichéd, is being a good person, a really good person. Not on paper, but genuinely. What matters is being conscious. Spirituality is a great little something to have in your top pocket. It gives you a whole lot of meaning and comfort; but so does having hobbies, jobs, families, pets, holidays. Wherever you find meaning is generally valid...with one proviso...you harm no one.

Spirituality is a trip, it's a pleasure, but is it what I'm here to discover? Not so much, I don't think. I'm here for the pleasures of the flesh and wonders of the mind. I'm here to get riled up whilst bra shopping and find ways to deal with those emotions. Spiritual living is guidance and warmth sitting at the heart of all that is. But does it really matter? No, not so much. It's like air to me, I need it, but I know it's there, I breathe it automatically, I need not think about it all the time, it remains there, and it doesn't ever leave.

22 November 2011
The joy of a good bra!

Oh my gosh. After weeks of weird boob pain – mainly extremely painful bouts of burning/stinging nipples – I have finally got a decent bra. It was purchased cheaper than a bottle of cheap wine in the local supermarket's 'for sale' section; the difference is immense, as indeed are the boobs!

Plus today I had not a single noticeable symptom; am I finally reaching the triumph of trimester two? Lots of energy – check. No sickness – check. Maybe so... Feeling good. Maybe I'm just on the up side of a hormonal swing, who cares, I'm riding it. Life is good, boobs are supported and I am smiling.

There was a noticeable difference in teaching my meditation class today. The last few weeks I hated it, as I felt so nauseous. There is nothing to throw off a peaceful mind like your pregnant mediation teacher puking… right! It was surely a case of too much 'vom' and not enough 'om'! Today I'm back to loving it! Though not sure how long that will last, I'm getting uncomfortable. Sitting crossed leg on the floor will not be an option for much longer.

I love being pregnant.

23 November 2011

I accidentally heard Cliff Richard crooning on the radio the other day. He was singing his hit, 'The Young Ones'. I listened closely and it drew me in. The song has been in my head ever since. Being Sir Cliff, the tone is mellow, so it's not been a nuisance, just a pleasant backing track as I go about my business. Indeed it has. It brought about some thoughts in me. I have always been 'The Young Ones'. I'm still (just about) the youngest generation of my family. At thirty-three I'm 'the kids'. Surely I'm amongst one of the first generation not forced to grow up age twenty-one. I'm a babied generation, encouraged to go to university; not for the education, but to spin youth out a little longer.

My parents seem to have got married and had kids because they were encouraged into adulthood. Throwing away their water wings before, perhaps, they were quite sure of their swimming ability. Whereas my generation have clung to the shallow ends, refusing to get bogged down in ceremony, commitment, responsibilities or ties. We have steadfastly remained 'The Young Ones'.

But of course that becomes stagnant and boring. Growing up,

in whatever format it comes, is an inevitability. This doesn't mean a magic formula should be enacted – i.e. marriage, kids, mortgage, move to the country. Oh no. I think that's where we get confused. Our prescribed notion of 'grown up' comprises the above elements in a way that is terrifying. It's like a dull and dire tick list of 'adult achievement'; and you don't get so much as a gold star once each box is ticked!

I think we are all ever so confused.

The line between young and old is too stark. We should go easy on ourselves, do what we want to do, in our own time – be it marriage or leading an expedition to uncover Atlantis. Being a grown up is not a task list. It's a state of mind. It's being conscious, aware, caring, concerned for your effect – on yourself and others. It's taken me a few years and three books to even think about that. And I'm glad I have, as Sir Cliff points out, we will soon be 'raising young ones of our own'.

Instead of holding crazily onto my youth, I'm willing to relinquish some of it's facets, though I hold dear to the good bits, the fun, the innocence, the curiosity, the sheer pleasure of being new. None of us are here long, so in hat respect we are all new. Adulthood is not an excuse to stagnate or rot. Because we are older we should not be inclined to hit a flat line. There is a balance to be struck. A fine wine when aged can still get you giddy. I intend to be a giddy adult, a giddy momma.

And so the wheel turns...

Onto another point I have been pregnantly pondering. Worry is such a waste of time. Worrying about worry, even more pointless. The upshot being I want to stop worrying about worrying.

In my latest therapy course class we practiced a technique whereby you embrace your negative emotions, really feel them deep inside, then you consider how you want to feel – the positive powerful emotions. You then switch between the bad and good feelings several times. After five or six attempts it is abundantly clear that 1) the negative feelings are weak – and perhaps a little stupid; and, 2) you are wholly capable of changing the way you think and feel at will; and so, therefore, you are a damned fool to yourself if you keep choosing the dark path.

So empowering. Mommas to be should all embark on a little self-improvement. We should all get to grips with our worries and fears so as not to bring up our little ones in a way that is fear led. We all owe it to our Poppyseeds to come into this life to a momma who has a clear, worry-free mind.

23 November 2011

Driving to my day job I felt particularly moved by Elton John's, 'Tiny Dancer' on the radio. Seems that all romantic songs are suddenly about my little baby. Little Poppyseed is a tiny, tiny dancer. Indeed, the first scan photo clearly shows him or her doing what can only be described as the 'Staying Alive' dance.

Also today, in a lovely coincidence, I received a bunch of Shamanic incenses from Sacred Valley Farm. These incenses are said to help with spiritual meditative journeying. The coincidence being that I had being thinking I really needed to do some more journeying. I am after all undergoing Shamanic training and last time I did a journey, I met the soul of my Poppyseed. I haven't really got an excuse now have I?

I keep getting this horrendous stinging breast pain...I may have mentioned it… Had a bout this morning. It only lasts about ten minutes but it a horrific ten minutes. When it happens I feel myself getting freaked out and upset. It really, really hurts. Really hurts. It totally takes me over when it occurs. It makes me want to cry.

Last time it happened it occurred to me that childbirth is going to be so much worse. Then I freaked out a little more. I'm blessed, as I've not had a lot of physical pain in my life. Never broken a bone or suffered a serious illness, not even as much as a nosebleed. It's all been a bit charmed.

I could rest on my laurels and expect an easy birth. However, I think maybe not. Now might be the right time to start practicing my hypnobirthing techniques. If I have to feel the pain, I must at least prepare for it. I don't want baba being born to a panic gripped, stressed crazed momma. If worst comes to worst I want to feel the pain and just be with it. Be with pain and bring forth life. Sounds so simple right? Roll on six months and we'll see how I go.

✡

24 November 2011
40-inch belly.

✡

25 November 2011
Feeling generally wonderful and hugely positive. The job that I have been frustrated by for several years is suddenly incredible and I'm enjoying it. Life is so pleasant. The little worries have dropped off and I don't care. What I mean is, I don't care about all the crap and nonsense. This leaves so much more space for happy feelings. Utterly blissful. Life is good.

Belly news. Still up and down. Every time I think it is appearing, it slinks back inside again. I'm really eating well. Not too much gluttony and I am keeping count so I know. A few meat cravings have come my way but very convincing fake burgers on gluten free buns, loads of ketchup and a hunk of cheese have soothed these. Delicious. Also loving oranges, apples and other fruits. Again delicious. It's so lovely to just eat and to not have any small guilt and worry of it sitting on my tummy – because it will anyway, and for all the right reasons.

25 November 2011

Decided to do a Shamanic journey. Within this, I was mentally visited by intense colors and a giant tree of life. Around the tree were dozens of people splashed with neon paint. I slipped under the roots of the tree and took a water slide down to fox's lair. Fox gave me advice, told me not to worry for the past as if it hadn't happened I would not be where I am now. Damn sound advice foxy.

26 November 2011

Waist 34-inch. Belly 39-inch. Lost an inch. No doubt because I am avoiding bread as it swells me up and makes me feel nasty. Pregnancy brings enough yuck as it is in terms of digestion-related issues. Toast is lovely, but an unproblematic tum is preferable right now.

The last thing I want in the entire world is for anyone to feel jealous of me. Today my friend admitted that me being pregnant did indeed make her a tad jealous.

This made me uncomfortable, because, for me, jealousy has a hostility to it, perhaps even a resentment; but she was very open and honest and I don't think this is how she meant it at all. She has wanted kids since forever and a recent love-split put paid to that for the time being. She will get there, I'm sure. Life can be a real bugger. But I guess we all have our paths, our circumstances to navigate and overcome.

27 November 2011
Had a very 'housie' day. Went to the gym in the morning, and then ate a 500 calorie chocolate croissant. I spent all afternoon sorting out drawers and cupboards. Didn't feel pregnant, not even once. Had a few back twinges and at one point got extremely hungry and devoured a bunch of buttery crumpets, but otherwise, business as usual.

Wondering over my still almost flat tummy, until I looked in the mirror and saw it was not so flat as I'd thought – though the croissant and crumpet bread party may be in part responsible. No matter what the cause of this newfound bump, it was most definitely a clear small protrusion. Had a dance around the living room with James and shook my stuff. Happy to report that belly is still small enough to not affect my centre of balance! Loving it, loving everything.

Took my happy vibe and burned some bad memories that I stumbled across (old diaries, letters etc) making way for good memories to be made. I recycled some other memories, as too much burning seems terribly wasteful. There is no need to dwell on the past or have the past inhabit my home in paper form. The past has officially gone to the winds.

I'm was just now out of the bath and drying off when something caught my eye, something was sticking out between my melon-like boobs. It was my tummy. Yep it never did that before! That's definitely new on me. Plus I need the toilet less – does this mean baby has moved upwards?

Had a nice night. Had a long phone chat with Helen an old friend from university. She has been through the mill lately, so we compared notes. It is always really inspiring to hear tales of people developing and growing through adversity. It's the only thing worth doing – living through hell and coming out better, stronger, and happier. Yes, that is the only option.

30 November 2011
When am I going to look properly pregnant I wonder? I keep thinking the bump has arrived, but, nope not yet, not really. Things have been pretty mundane this week; James has been working hard putting up walls in the baby's room. I have been feeling pretty normal. I spent Sunday cleaning and clearing out space with lashings of energy.

Everyone at work is striking today; it's a big walk out. I couldn't bring myself to do it. James is working himself silly, and me sitting on my ass peeing overtime money up the wall is not something I am happy to do. I'm not wasting money that could go on our baby... This is not very community focused I know, but right now, my priorities are with my immediate life. I can't see poor James struggling whilst I waste money. My loyalty in this instance is with us. Not going to work would have felt deeply disrespectful to him. He was fine if I did strike, but it didn't feel right. So here I am sat at work, writing up my diary…In my lunch break, of course.

1 December 2012
Waist 34.5-inch, Belly 39.5-inch.

Had a mad, lovely dream last night. Dreamt I was driving to my American Grandparents old farmhouse in Kentucky. It was just like how it used to be; I felt a perfect sense of peace and comfort as we pulled up into the garage. Poignant because I'll never go there again as they've moved to a new home. Baby will never go there and that makes me a little sad. So many happy memories. A big bliss of 'happy'.

Then I dreamt that my Grandparents took us to a field behind the house to hitch a lift on a private plane. The pilots explained that it doesn't work like that. I was relieved. I didn't want to get on the tiny plane. Also dreamt we were all locked out of the farmhouse. Hanging round in the fields with the animals. Crazy but cool, animals make good company.

2 December 2012
Today I was accused of having 'preg head'! Probably not wholly untrue. This results from yesterday when we had a meeting at work and I accused the senior management team of being like George W Bush and his cronies. I then continued to rant on about how the staff survey was propaganda. I mean I really went on and on and on. Not just the once either. I raised the issue once, then again later in the meeting. I turned into some kind of crazed conspiracy theorist. I may have even mentioned the devil and evil forces. I can't quite remember, it's all a blur. I was possessed with the spirit of David Icke, but without his oratory skills.

Normally I rarely speak in meetings at work. My point being, that at the time I felt strongly, but the comparison was probably a little extreme. Looking back, I'm not quite sure why I felt so strongly… I think I was whipped into a frenzy by other people's feelings and instead of sitting back and watching the clock, I just let rip. In retrospect, I don't even agree with what I said…It was borderline hysterical. At the time though I was so righteous and believed I had the management sussed!

I also gave someone the finger yesterday whilst driving. This is so, so unlike me, and so the opposite of spiritual. In my defense, I was letting a little old man cross the road in front of my car. The car behind me started beeping at me. It just made me see red. I never get road rage. But then again I never start spouting about George W Bush and the illuminati before.

I wouldn't say I'm angry, more passionate, though perhaps on the crazy side of passionate right now. I don't feel so worried about what people think or feel. Particularly when it comes to ethics. I refuse to run over old people. If I think senior management are feeding us propaganda then it is my place to revolt – though maybe I should sleep on it first!

I have preg-head and I am a revolutionary!

2 December 2012

There is someone I'm struggling to forgive.

And yet I am spiritual. I preach forgiveness and I know that releasing my pain would be healing. I too am human and here I have a stumbling block. My anger and frustration feels pertinent, natural, and righteous. Part of me does not want to release it.

Though inside of my anger, I wonder if the person I'm mad at has become a scapegoat for all manner of things. I am focusing all my hurt onto that person. I know I'm doing that, and it's too easy to carry on doing it. At the very same time, I know that all the wondrous things in my life wouldn't have happened had that person, and all the pain they caused, not have occurred. It all needed to happen. Yet I have this residual anger and hurt towards them. I'd like it to go away. I think I need to work on this.

It's been ten minutes since I wrote the above confession and I feel I have moved massively. Just pondering on the whole situation and writing about it seems to have caused an inner shift. Suddenly I'm stuck between wishing to scream bloody fury at the person, and desiring strongly to make some kind of peace.

The peace I need to make is perhaps not with the person as an individual, but it is within myself. I don't want to be friends, but forgiveness suddenly seems to be more about my welfare than anything else. In keeping myself in a place of indignant fury, am I not just making myself feel bad? Am I not just sprawling out a situation that I could put to bed and get on with my life? What I must do is let it out, let it go, release it and all that other hippy shit.

I truly don't believe people are 'bad'. They do what they do and often they believe what they are doing is correct. In my heart of hearts, I know that what hurt me was not about me. It rarely is. This certain person helped their self and I was hurt as a side effect. Yes they could and should have behaved differently, thought before they acted… But I know their selfish actions were not done to spite me, they were done despite me.

No one meant to cause me pain; they only found a way to deal with their life in a way that seemed necessary at the time. All things happen for a reason, there are no mistakes. I must just keep telling myself that.

Probably we have all hurt others when thinking that we are helping ourselves. The junkie is feeding an immediate personal need not trying to destroy his family. The burglar steals to make ends meet, not because he wants to plague a household with terror. The bully hurts others essentially to make himself feel better. The bitch makes nasty comments because something is missing in her soul. The mother spanks the child to make them see sense, and to try to show how that child can be better. We all act in self-defense all the time, other people's pain is not usually our goal, but the soothing of our own pain usually is. This doesn't mean that bad behavior; burglary, spanking or bitching is tolerable. It just means we can be at peace with it, if we realize that it came from a place that was not vengeful against us. If we can see that more often than not, pain caused to us, is not personal. For me, it means I can see a meaning within the madness, and get on with my life anger free.

This diary entry has brought me a lot of closure. I've gone from angry to remarkably philosophical. Pen and paper can be the best therapy.

My conclusion is this; this person was instrumental not in wrecking my life, but in helping whip up the chaos that was much needed. This chaos played a part in bringing life to where it is now and helping to bring a beautiful Poppyseed to my belly.

I wouldn't change it for the world.

3 December 2012
Last night I went out for dinner with Roisin and Reina and their other halves, Brian and Dave. We had a lengthy conversation about avoiding cats defecating in your garden. Apparently there are amazing sonic devices that can really help prevent this.

Over the years our conversations have steered across what to wear at weekends, drinking, dating, dumping, moving in, mortgages and now children – plus the cherry on the cake that is cat poop. A sure fire sign you are ready to be parents!

There was much reminiscing about drunken times. Lots of stories were told. I remember very little of them. Which, trust me, says more about my youthful alcohol intake than it does about my memory.

Ah, the excesses of youth.

Reina commented that at least we were never 'out of control'. I pointed out that she speaks for herself on that one as I feel I really truly was on occasions. Examples are cropping up in my mind immediately. I can't bear to put them to paper…I have definitely been out of control, and not always whilst I was under the influence. I have been out of control and sober too. Before my spirituality took hold, my mind was a mad house and this mad house wasn't fun. The partying I indulged in to avoid thinking too much, certainly helped. But I too, like my ex-friend in the last entry, have been a bit of an arse in my time. I've acted out of self-interest and hurt other people. Happily, I don't miss any of it. The corner that I've turned does not allow for much backward glancing.

Today was wonderful. It was the day of my therapy course and the synchronicity of it all was marvelous. It turns out that today's subjects were anger and forgiveness. The magic of non-coincidence never fails to amaze me. I know this course is changing me for the better, and with yesterdays self-counseling about forgiveness, combined with the forgiveness done on the course, it seems my higher self and the universe are conspiring to make me a better, happier mum-to-be.

On another note, I was moved to deep sadness by a story on the news of an abused baby. I know that bad stuff happens, but this really got to me. Now I have a Poppyseed sprouting inside of me tales of abuse are harder to stomach.

My prayers and love to that poor little child. Angels, if you are reading this make it better for him, make him strong and protect him.

Love and light to all the innocents.

5 December 2012

Well, it's all been a bit cerebral recently. It's time for a physical round up. I am generally exhausted. I've had two days off in four weeks and spent those days doing house stuff. It feels that when I have 'downtime' I literally collapse, watch trash TV, eat something and fall into bed.

Whilst many say I should slow down and enjoy the pregnancy, I can't do this because I'm not, not enjoying it. I positively am enjoying it. Whatever I'm doing, and wherever I do it, the pregnancy is with me and makes it all the more meaningful. I will slow down when I need to, but I do what I do out of choice, and baby comes with me. Every moment has baby at the heart of it, whether I'm ranting in work meetings or lounging in the bath. Whether I move fast or slow, I breathe and exist for baby. I don't need to slow down to enjoy anything.

I'm still looking only vaguely pregnant. I'm sixteen weeks this week and apparently Poppyseed will double in size now. So I'm preparing to wave goodbye to the last of my normal wardrobe. My breasts are huge and still suffer appalling outbursts of burning pain. At night, when I get really tired, I become so fidgety that my body pushes me up to bed. It's a fearsome mess that cannot be ignored and must be obeyed. I noticed yesterday that lying on my tummy feels odd now. As though I'm lying on top of a small beach ball.

I think I feel flutters – little pops and bubbles in my belly. I felt it once in bed, once in my class this weekend and once just now.

I spent some time meditating with baby last night. I mentally cleansed all my chakras and then cleansed the baby's chakras too, I'm sure baby won't object. Was sweet to have a few moments chilling with Poppyseed.

Whilst I've been on my course all weekend James has spent all weekend finishing putting walls on the baby's bedroom. He's worked hard and done a fantastic solo job. We spent last night daubing silly comments and Reiki symbols all over the new walls. Lord knows what the plasterer will make of it all! Nirvana smiley faces sat next to powerful Reiki symbols. This pretty much sums up what baby is letting him/her self in for. Rock and Soul baby! Rock and Soul.

James was telling me today about how starkly peoples' attitudes towards kids have changed now the initial congratulations have worn off. On first learning we were pregnant his work mates patted him on the back and advised him that having kids was the best thing they ever did. Some months down the line, this parental camaraderie has given way to sheer negativity. With one colleague advising that we wrap our bundle of joy up and leave it in the woods. Alongside the ever-classy retrospective 'If I had my time again I never would...'

My stance on this is simple – life is hard. Many people live everyday as though life is happening to them. Such people will always find ways to blame their 'unique' misery on others. They blame their parents, their partner, their boss, their kids, their dog, their friend, the government and of course the weather.

Do these people ever stop to consider that maybe it is no-one's fault and that they choose their lives and therefore ultimately have control over how they feel? Yes, a wayward teen or crying baba may be stressful, heartbreaking even, but your misery is your own and you should choose to hold it.

Life is hard and that is that. I choose a family and all that this entails. I do so consciously, and with a heart full of faith that the good will outweigh the bad. And if the bad overtakes the good, as it tends to do sometimes, I will hope that the growth and learning for all involved, eventually overtakes any misery.

Dear Poppyseed,
Hey there little child – I'm so tired tonight. Momma's been busy, too busy; she is going to slow down now and take more time out to send you some loving vibes. Hope all is well in belly-town and please excuse me keep poking around your watery home. I can't help it; I hope I may catch a feel of you!

I think I felt you bubble a few times; I'm looking forward to more of that.

Love and belly kisses

Mum.

8 December 2011
Baby is only a tiny 4mm as of yesterday. Waist 34-inch. Bump 40-inch.

What a total palaver. Today heralded a massive reminder of my imminent uselessness. Took James to see Motley Crew and Def Leppard for an early birthday present. On the way into the gig I realized I desperately needed a wee. I needed a wee way, way, way more than is usual. I had a concerned feeling I may have a terrible accident. This was new to me. I have been desperate for a wee before, but never to the point of feeling like the liquid may drop out of me at any given moment. Never before have I felt such a huge pressure and lack of control over what may happen next to my bodily functions.

Upon arrival at the venue, I left James to get us drinks and I dashed off to the toilet. In my haste, and perhaps due to a number of factors – slippery floor, worn down heels, hurriedness, new centre of gravity, loose ligaments – I took a massive fall. I landed on all fours in front of a few dozen hard-core, longhaired rockers; my legs splayed out and face an ever-deepening shade of red.

No one came to my aid, so after an indeterminate time in doggy position I got myself up and fled, humiliated, into the toilets. I flung myself into a cubicle and promptly burst into tears. I do not remember the last time I fell over – probably it was when I was a child. This was a gross reminder of the fact that it's not the pain that causes the tears, but the overwhelming shock and humiliation.

I sobbed for some time. Those hot, unstoppable tears that stream down your face flooded me. The horrid choking feeling and tight chest that comes with real emotion accompanied this. Once I regained some form of composure and put my glasses on (so that I might be in disguise) I ventured out to find James. Then on sighting him, I burst into tears again. He was a sweetie, he took me off to the corner, gave me a few cuddles, and a lecture on sensible shoes. Together we trundled off for a night of Rock and for me a soothing hot chocolate.

This was an interesting reminder of my vulnerability. One that was probably quite timely. It's all very well preaching the virtues of the soul, but when your fancy shoes meet polished floor, spirituality goes out the window. When one's face greets the floor and all dignity is lost, it is time to reassess. So having written two books with 'High Heeled' in the title, I now officially relinquish all heels, even kitten heels and embrace the future. My future is flat.

9 December 2011

I've had just the busiest few days. I've barely stopped and I am exhausted. Tonight James is out and for the first time in ages I'm alone, chilling out on the couch with Jimi cat sat on my knee.

Suddenly as if from nowhere my stomach moved!

There is no shadow of a doubt in my mind that it was anything but baby. Even Jimi cat woke up and took a look! Magic. I can say for sure that this was the most definite first movement. What a beautiful thing – just baby, Jimi and me.

This kick, punch or somersault was not how I expected it to feel. I thought a baby movement would feel as though it were deep within struggling to get out. But this was a shallow, on the surface feeling. It was as if something popped on the edge of my belly, just under the flesh and made the outside wobble and move. How incredible.

11 December 2012

Today was a lovely day. Woke at nine but didn't get out of bed until about half eleven. I have developed a love of nothingness – just staring into space, hand on belly, thinking, mind wandering. Same again tonight, James went to bed early and I laid on the sofa looking around, breathing, thinking, hand on belly. Nothing boring about it. Just loved the peace, quiet and safety.

15 December 2012

I have been somewhat distracted from pregnancy by everyday life. First up have been Christmas decorations, secondly stress over the house being upside down due to a desk. The desk saga has been rolling on months with no end in sight, and has upped James's stress levels a little too high for comfort.

He is having a desk built in his studio. Until it's built, the studio is unworkable. For one reason and another, it hasn't happened yet. It's no ones fault, but it is unfortunate. It's been a year of monumental change but this desk situation is like a stubborn blackhead ruining an otherwise flawless finish. I know it will get sorted out and my spiritual inclinations are currently poured into the deep hope that a desk related miracle occurs... and soon!

Just booked in for an early baby gender scan. Got an amazing cheap deal on a voucher website. This is so stupidly exciting. We will find out the sex next Tuesday and surprise the parents with it on Christmas Day. Makes a family Christmas well worth its weight in gold. Five sleeps until lad or lass is confirmed.

16 December 2012

I am so cozy today, wearing James's jeans, jumper and leather jacket, making a very comfy 'in between' size option. It's nice being wrapped up in Daddy.

James is out on his Christmas work's do tonight. So it is just me, bump and the cats watching a bit of TV. I felt the baby tickle my tummy. Then, when I got in bed, a hard round lump formed on the left side of my stomach. I felt overwhelmed with love. Baby said goodnight. Time to shut off now and let my heartbeat carry me and baby to the land of nod...

17 December 2012

Woke up feeling fresh today despite being woken at 2am by James returning from his work's Christmas do. He was happy, smiley drunk and I told him about the baby moving.

Realized today, as I realize often, that in spite of the downsides to pregnancy – like exhaustion or burning boobs I actually love it. It's an incredible experience, the absolute best. Plus I've never been healthier. Normally by December I would have succumbed to at least one or two bad colds that knock me off my feet, but nothing yet. Feeling really well so the baby-bump hormones, healthy eating and pregnancy vitamins must be protecting me from the lurgies of winter!

I'm still enjoying my new love of sitting in silence and staring into space. Whilst my body is tired my mind is doing fun things. Every night brings a barrage of intriguing and entertaining dreams. Last night, in between dreams of painting and solving riddles, I dreamt that a doctor announced to me I was having a boy. Three days till an actual gender scan, I will soon know if that dream is a vision of the future or not!

20 December 2012

Waist 36 inches Belly 42 inches – up 2 inches!

Today is the day that, baby willing, we learn the gender of little Poppyseed. We are both so exited, though impending parenthood is bringing up a few 'issues'. Last night James was keen to talk about how we should never argue in front of our child. Then went on to criticize my domestic skills. I freely admit that I'm not the tidiest person, but nor am I dirty. I just have a higher tolerance for the 'lived in' look. We almost argued on the subject but skillfully both managed to keep our cool. This pregnancy lark is gifting us with a higher degree of tolerance and better listening skills, at least for now. So whilst the domestics might have brought on an attack of grumbling, tonight it did not. Soulful living is a beautiful thing, but meditation and positive thought won't clean the dishes. Bring on the marigolds!

On a spiritual note just as James and I left the house, circling over our heads was a lone, quacking duck. Not sure as yet what this may be symbolic of, but if birds are the symbols I believe they are, then this certainly meant something. Maybe ducky was simply heralding in a new era with little Mr or Mrs Baby.

We are having a girl!
I am so happy. I had almost convinced myself it was a boy, but when the lady with the ultrasound said, and I quote, 'this baby is a girl' I promptly burst into happiness tears.

I knew James wanted a girl and perhaps that's why I was so convinced it could be a boy. Just to be sure we were prepared for either and to balance things out. I'm all doey-eyed and happy now. I'm also really sleepy as the three-hour wait between work and going for the scan was stressful... Too many of our friends have gone for scans only to hear terrible tragic news. But happily all is well. We have a chunky girl child growing in my uterus. Fabulous, fabulous, fabulous.

Before becoming pregnant ,and in moments of broodiness over the years, I always envisioned myself with a little girl. In the past her name was Dakota. But for now her name is… well I'll keep that to myself.

I just want to experience this feeling forever. I feel like quitting everything, just to be at one with my little baby girl. I could put down this pen and never write another word.

Dear Poppyseed,
Well hello little girl. Mummy is so pleased to know you a little more. I can't tell you the fantasies I've had of you being in my life. Me and my little gal pal, crossing oceans, climbing mountains,

sharing secrets, being best friends and holding hands through the years. People say you can't be friends with your children. That is their opinion. I am your friend no matter what, even if you find me embarrassing and uncool when I kiss you at the school gates. I'm your friend when you throw a tantrum. I'm your friend when you become all consumed with your first love. I'm your friend when perhaps that is the last thing you want. I'm your friend when life gets in the way and you'd rather be doing anything else than hanging around with your old mum! Little chica, some people also say that we come into this world alone. You don't. You come in with me waiting to catch you. I'm forever your friend little girl.

21 December 2012
A day on and I'm still so happy. I have spoken to a few friends who all remember my dalliance with the imaginary Dakota. Given the events of the past few years the fantasy of my little girl and me subsided; but it used to be very real and tangible. And now a few years later it is true and it's a surprise because I'd been certain I was having a boy. Which makes it the best surprise ever. I'm still gushing, I'm pink and excited.

22 December 2012
All change. I may have neglected to mention my work situation until now. Poppyseed has proven an utter distraction. As well as being an author, I have for a while held down a normal old day job too. I started the job way before the books were conceived and I've been there for seven years now. Of late, we have been facing an office closure and potential redundancy. Happily, my department is being enabled to work from home, which means at

least we keep our jobs. But it is now the last days and faces are disappearing from the office never to return in the same capacity. People who have become the fabric of our lives are all vanishing to their lonesome spare rooms to work on files in between hanging out the washing and petting their cats.

Seven years seems like a good time for a natural end, but it's still hard to leave a buzzing environment for one where the only buzz is that of your modem. I'm really over the moon however, because working from home means being with baby more. I have childcare in the form of Grandma's and I won't have to leave to go to an office, whilst leaving baby without my presence all day long. That must be so heartbreaking. It's all worked out rather well. Plus, after I return from Maternity leave, I have a three-month grace period working from home. If I don't like it, or it doesn't work for me, I get to take redundancy. It's not a bad situation to be in. I'm very lucky.

I had a strange, but oddly welcome, financial situation today. I received a letter from my car loan people saying that the final amount was due immediately. Well a Happy Christmas to you too. I had forgotten all about this 'final payment' many moons ago. Happily we had squirreled away the exact right amount and with last month's overtime I scraped the payment with sufficient left for mince pies. Unfortunately, all of my buffer money was swallowed up in one shot. Including the secret stash I had earmarked for Poppyseed. On the up side, the car is now mine and despite empty savings I feel as though I've been spring-cleaned. A big debt has been paid off by money that was otherwise gathering dust. There is room for growth here. Dusty money is not an attractor of abundance. This situation feels right.

Now that the money has gone to a valid home I feel ready to accumulate fresh funds. There is a spiritual lesson here; don't hoard or hang on to money energy that could be used quite successfully elsewhere. Savings are great, but not when there is debt to be paid. We have a financial clean slate for a new year.

And for the first time ever I own my car outright. Perhaps now I ought to clean it...

James went to visit his best friend Neil today and I had my first alone time in weeks. Scrolling through my phones baby related application, I decided to zip all the way down to April/May. An entry on April 25 2012 stated that my baby would be full term and could be born any time from there onward – so in essence, Poppyseed could be here in four months. I'm barely showing, yet in four months I could be ready to pop.

How ironic that at the gym two people remarked how slim I was. Not sure where that came from? I use the gym mirrors as a true indicator of how big my stomach is. The mirrors at home seem to be on the skinny side. In the gym mirrors I wouldn't say I look slim. If I suck in I look period bloated, maybe a bit pot bellied. If I let it all hang loose, then I guess I look either very bloated or a little pregnant.

I guess I'm half way there and suddenly one lengthy and expansive four months seems like a drop in the ocean.

This makes me nervous. I'm not ready yet. I'm enjoying the preparations too much. I'm not sure either if I'm nervous for labor, for being a parent, for the real expansion of my tummy, for fear of not being ready or all those things combined and perhaps some other ones that haven't yet sprung to mind. I'm having a mid-term wobble. A very civilized, very quiet, very unemotional, but very real wobble!

Bedtime now, perhaps by morning the wobble will wobble off! Tomorrow is my last day in the office ever, so many changes in such a short space of time. Wow. Goodnight.

29 December 2012

Christmas has been a funny old time. It's heralded moments of joy, but on the other hand, it's had its fair share of stressful. James has been pulling his hair out with frustration getting the baby's room ready, after finishing the studio (Mabbey Road – 12 months in the making). We have had a plasterer in since Boxing Day (more fool us), and we have spent much time cleaning up after him. James has gone from upbeat and positive, to vexed and singing the blues, with good reason. I love him to bits but when his balance is out of whack, he is harder to live with.

This is not helped by me feeling anxious about impending motherhood. I'd be lying if I said that the four-month window to potential baby time isn't freaking me out somewhat. In four months time everything changes. Everything. I really am looking forward to some of those changes and the soulful experience of motherhood, but right now, I'm also slightly worried about what I'm entering into.

First up to go will be my total autonomy and independence. I won't be able to do what I want, whenever I want. Not that I'm hugely impetuous, or liable to flit off doing things. But I guess I won't have the option. Or at least I'll have less of an option.

Perhaps this isn't such a huge issue. I'll embrace my new limitations.

Second, I'm waving goodbye to my youth. I don't care how much of a yummy mummy I may aspire to be, there are things I'll never, ever do again. Once you're a parent you can't be irresponsible, crazy or wild. Not that I am inclined in those ways much these days. But having a baby is the final nail in the coffin that was my irresponsibility. No bad thing perhaps... Whilst I may be losing my culturally embedded version of youth, I will, no doubt, embrace my inner child. That's a fair swap. I'll take it.

Thirdly physical trauma and changes loom. James mentioned that breastfeeding can wreak havoc with your boobs. I don't think he is actually correct about this, but my vanity kicked in, and a little panic may well have risen in my gut. But let's be honest, I'm thirty-three, my boobs are only going south anyway. Swapping them and other physical assets, to meet the baby love of my life, is something I can deal with.

So my three fears, on inspection, are not so scary. In fact they seem rather shallow. They don't stand up to scrutiny. Poppyseed beats them all hands down. Happy days, moving into motherhood looks suddenly brighter. Bring on the saggy boobs and restrictions; they are nothing, nothing at all. Life is about love and that is what I will embrace. Love, saggy bits and schedules are the future!

Dear Poppyseed,
On Christmas Day we went for lunch with your Grandma Becky, Grandma Karen, Nana Bev and Grandpa Tony M. You are honored to have so many Grandmas. You have a Grandma Aileen too. It's a veritable clan of women who will guard you and love you beyond yourself.

Anyway, as Daddy and I know you are a girl, we decided to keep this information to ourselves. We waited until everyone arrived for Christmas lunch and then we presented them with a pink envelope each. Inside the envelopes were, 'It's a Girl' cards. To say the response was emotional was an understatement. I'm sure everyone would have been equally happy had you been a boy. But I hope that knowing you are a girl means all your Grandparents feel closer to you. Plus they can now put a name to you and start planning your summer wardrobe!

The first of many happy Christmases we will share with you.

Love, Mum

1 January 2012
Well thank goodness for that, a fresh shiny new year. 2011 was chaotic and at times felt dangerous. Early on in the year it felt

that life as I knew it, was on thin ice. Life was precarious as James and I pulled ourselves out of a dark and dingy time, but, as ever, my belief in chaos bringing about sense prevailed. I believe that we need the hard times; they literally make us who we are. If the harsher events of 2010/11 hadn't happened the ground would not have been prepared for this new life, for Poppyseed. So there's no point postulating, cursing and thinking back negatively. 2011 did a job, and it did it well. The fact it often felt horrible is irrelevant.

From a spiritual perspective I have nothing but praise and thanks for the pain I endured. From a human perspective, goodbye and good riddance. Happy New Year!

There are many spiritual theories about 2012. Could it be the end of the world? A raising of consciousness? I prefer the latter and I'd vote for that if votes were enabled. The world has been a hectic, chaotic place of late, reflected in my own life, I've felt the pain, and I've seen chaos in the life of friends, in society and across global events. What comes next is liable to be more of the same. Followed, I hope, by much enlightenment, and hopefully, hopefully, hopefully planet earth will become a kinder more soul-fulfilling place to live. I'll do what I can to add to that and I'll be sure to give Poppyseed a foundation in soulfulness. I will rest assured that my life will reflect and propagate soulful loveliness. That is enough...right?

Back to the daily human side of things. The house is upside down; we still have a plasterer in doing the baby's bedroom walls. He is the messiest bugger I ever met; on his breaks (which he has a lot of) I swear he is smoking pot. We have spent three days cleaning up after him and making more cups of tea than I feel is necessary. Every day has involved full on deep cleans, just to make the house bearable, just to repeat again over and over.

We are exhausted with it and James and I had a massive row over a dustsheet, which was nothing more than ridiculous. He said he told me to put it over the computer. I say he simply mentioned there was a dustsheet and must have imagined he told me where to put it! Irrespective of what was said, my own reaction in this argument went shamefully against my spiritual inclinations. However, I choose to forgive myself and move on. Funny how these little domestic bickerings can feel so damned significant at the time!

On top of this, Molly cat has had a poorly paw and has clearly been attention seeking. My rabbits appear to be having issues amongst themselves as the two youngest are locked in some kind of leadership battle. I attempted to mediate but thought better of it when I got badly scratched up. It's their problem and I'll let them figure it out.

I've been in touch with a Doula. I want to explore natural birthing and hypnobirthing a little more. I'll await her response before I think about this any further.

Last night was a sober New Year's Eve for me. Went out to a bar for a few hours, home just before midnight, in time for a kiss in front of the TV as Big Ben chimed in 2012. I stayed up with James until nearly four in the morning, a huge achievement, helped only by indulging in a massive lie in the previous day. Around three in the morning we did some experimenting with lying down positions and James felt his first kick from his daughter. Beautiful moment and a happy 2012 to him! So this is it. The year of my baby, her birth and life already looks brighter. 2012, I love you already.

1 January 2012 ctd…
I chose an animal card to represent the New Year. I got Butterfly. Butterfly represents transformation, gestation, and change. It is our life reset. Perfect.

I also wrote our letter to the universe. We do this every year and have done for a few years. Usually we do it on New Years Eve whilst slightly tipsy. This year it was late and I was definitely sober. I wrote it, James burnt it, sure there's a cliché in there somewhere – what woman creates, man destroys...

This felt so potent this year with Poppyseed on the way. The idea of burning it means you can't keep checking the results against what was hoped for. Instead you make your wishes and allow the universe to be creative in interpretation. The universe always is, and I would never expect anything less. So here is hoping that cosmic forces go our way this year.

1 January 2012 ctd ctd…

I just found out that my friend Elly killed herself on New Years Eve, yesterday. Elly was my boss for a little while and was a close friend of my best mate, Roisin. She has been depressed a long while, maybe forever. Though I never saw that side to her. I only ever saw the excitable, fun-loving, hilarious, cocktail mixing side. Whilst I didn't know her hugely well, I knew her a little and it's surprising how a little knowledge can still leave a hole. She was a fun woman. The funniest train journey I ever had in my life involved her. You had to be there, but trust me, it was pure hilarity. She was an animal lover, like me. She was a sweet gal, but of course I believe she goes on... I hope she's okay wherever she is. 2012 is poorer without her.

2nd January 2012

I've been thinking a lot about inspiration. My mind has been turning inward and all manner of life situations have received my attention. Inspiration is often hard to find in the bleakness of winter, particularly after the lights of Christmas and fireworks of New Year have gone out, but if you look for it, you will find it. Even when you have to look extra hard.

Today's inspiration was found within the backdrop of Elly's very sad death. I have giggled to myself several times today as I revisited in my mind the train journey we took home from Reina's hen do in London. It was without doubt one of those classic life moments, and the funniest train journey I will ever expect to take, ever. We laughed and laughed and the women on the next table thanked us when they left because they too laughed and laughed. And the seventeen-year-old boy who was stuck at our table, tried to stifle his laughter as if he weren't listening, but in the end, he laughed and laughed too. London to Leicester on the laughter-line! Quite simply I'll never forget it.

In a way Elly's death holds its own little glimmer of inspiration. Death forces you to dig deep into what you have, into life, into living. With that shadowing everything, life starts to look brighter. The little things become easier to appreciate. There is sadness in death, but inspiration in a life lived, in the memories made and in the fact that the living can find a way to continue with a new found appreciation of things, all things, anything.

Ellen was a force to be reckoned with, she was zany, fun, hilarious and generous. Rather than grieve her death, it is for me to reconcile it, absorb it, and to be there for my friend who it has devastated. To do this I remember the good times, and that damned brilliant train journey.

Today was also the day James and I did our first bit of shopping for our little girl. Now I'm not a lover of shopping, not at all, but today it felt good, even on a rammed busy bank holiday retail park. Today the sun was sparkling on the tarmac and this home of commercial madness, seemed welcoming and warm. We were shopping for our home and for our little baby, and in this was great joy. All my shopping qualms aside, it was beautiful. What can I say...death can weave its effects in funny ways, and for me it has brought about a new perspective.

Today I found something twinkling and wonderful somewhere between a new life and a sad death. I found a perspective that saw me smiling more often because life is short and every moment is deeply valuable. A perspective that allowed me to let things be as they are, not to question, not to worry, to relax, to care for those around me and to be a good friend, a good partner, a good mother. Death brings new perspective like nothing else in this world. Except perhaps new life... Death and Life, the two levelers of human kind, the two things that make us real and that can offer the truest perspective we might ever experience.

Dear Poppyseed,
You have my permission, nay my encouragement to just give it up, get back to your roots and be human. So many people on a soulful path set themselves up to a very high standard. Perhaps sometimes a wholly unrealistic standard, one that has them setting themselves up to fail. I know I have in the past provided myself with a list of 'Divine Living Rules' that I pretty much failed at. In this failure I balked at myself, unsure of where my life stood.

Let's be straight on this, you do not lose your spirituality, your spirit or your divinity by doing anything at all. Those things are permanent fixtures of your soul, baby. Spirit and soul is your birthright, it's your pre-birth and afterlife right too! So if you indulge in gossip, swear at your Mom, insult an elderly person, get drunk, curse, think negatively, overreact, overindulge, fight with your friend, forget to say thank you or any other such horrendous sin, then heck I say, don't worry. Your soul is going nowhere. It is you.

The thing about this life is that it is where we are. We are meant to be human for a reason. We are meant to run up against our own fallibility's and failures and feel irksome and dirtied, muddy, rude, crude, lewd, tattooed - whatever!

There is the whole concept too about learning, growing and making good from our mistakes. Because I also strongly believe that there are no true mistakes. Never, ever, ever. Mistakes are opportunities by another name. Which is all very relevant and important, but right now I don't want to talk about that. I want to talk about the grime and the grit that will get you through life. That stuff makes you who you are. Because that stuff is really, very cool.

Every single bloody-minded move you make, for good, bad or worse has happened for a reason. If you learn from it then great, but if not, you also have to accept what you did and move on. Life is a difficult taskmaster and not a one of us is perfect. Not a one. Be sure of that my baby, because it makes the days and the chaos fly by us easier.

You are human. You are human not because it is your job to ascend to the heavens as soon as possible. But because, for whatever reason, your soul wanted to get it's hands dirty, it wanted to get up to it's knees, no, it's waist in mud. Being human, even being naughty can be fun. It all serves a purpose. If I hadn't been naughty in my time I would never have written my books, I wouldn't be me. I wouldn't have a damned thing to say for myself.

So be naughty, be neglectful, be silly, accept your hang-ups as a sheer result of your flesh and blood, and own your weaknesses as they can add up to one great big strength over time. Allow yourself to get muddy in the mess of human life. Get muddy and wallow it.

You are human for a reason sweetpea. Whatever else you do make the effort to be the human that you are. Love and forgive that human, show that human a good time! Embrace your mistakes and hold them proud in your heart. There is method in the madness darling. Trust me, I'm very much a human too.

Love from your Mum

4 January 2012

So far this year is pretty mellow, other than hearing next door's poorly kids vomiting all is well. A taste of things to come; sick children, most excellent…

I started working from home in the day job yesterday. Truly loving it. I feel so much more freedom. I can do bits of housework as I wander around, visit the gym at lunch, and hang out with the cats and bunnies. What's not to love?

Today I have started a blog on my website all about being inspired. It's a thirty-day feat of blogging endurance. I am feeling that…as ever…I may have taken too much on. Since discovering what I love to do (writing) I have developed bad habits of working too hard. This never used to be a problem!

I'm so busy with a full time job, writing books, spewing out blogs, book promotion for me and other authors, editing, publishing with my imprint Soul Rocks, articles for magazines, occasional tarot readings and weekly meditation classes; all this whilst trying also to have a life, see friends and spend time with James. I guess when baby arrives some of this may have to go…

I did a pregnancy exercise DVD last night. It was remarkably hard considering the DVD was some pretty basic squat type things. Not sure if my muscles have atrophied, despite visiting the gym lots, or perhaps it's just normal in pregnancy to be a putrid weakling. I intend to do that DVD more often. I want to be strong giving birth and if a few lousy squats and leg raises help, then so be it.

Today is also the start of my twentieth week pregnant. I'm halfway baked and I'm certainly feeling it. Bending over is a whole new experience that leaves me feeling about eighty years old. But what the heck, Miss Poppyseed has my permission to make herself at home. And if that means making me less than comfortable, then I will deal with it.

As for Poppyseed herself... I feel a need to connect more, but also feel a little daft singing or talking aloud to my bump. Not only is my mental songbook shockingly low on material, but also my heart is not always in it. I do intend to play her music and rub her through my belly wall that much is simple and easy. The rubbing comes naturally of course; I do that without even thinking. This diary is also a way of communicating. I believe Poppyseed's soul is more aware of what's going on than the physical Poppyseed in my belly right now. So I'll take the combo approach, I'll sing, chant, stroke and play music and I will make an effort to feel good so that she gets lots of calm, happy vibes and hormones. I'll also connect to her spirit through this diary and through holding her consistently in my thoughts. Poppyseed, baby girl, I'm sending you love right now.

6 January 2012

Just went to yoga at my gym. It wasn't pregnancy yoga but the teacher kindly modified it for me. Oh my, do I feel pregnant. And all of those mirrors in the gym made me realize I'm looking pretty damned pregnant too. There is no confusing this bump for bloat anymore! Inspite of my gaining size, I still really love to exercise, I feel it's so important to me. My workout routine is more regular than it ever was as a non-pregnant person and I intend to keep it that way.

At the end of the yoga class a particular position made baby go crazy. It felt as though she was doing her own set of yogic asana inside me. It was the strongest set of movements I have ever felt, so strong in fact that I was briefly concerned. For a split second I thought somehow the yoga had harmed her. But she soon settled down to a gentle bubble. I believe I'm growing myself a little yogi!

7 January 2012
Today I started to over think the whole baby situation. My neighbor's poorly children brought this about by crying and vomiting most of the week. We have thin walls here, and their retching and tearfulness was consistent. I felt so sorry for the parents. In turn I felt sorry for myself as a future parent. It brought about a whole unexpected set of 'What if…' What if…I don't like being a mum? What if…I resent my crying child? What if…I can't cope? I was tossing and turning in bed, contemplating all of this and eventually I fell back to sleep. I dreamt I was holding my baby girl, gazing into her eyes and declaring them the most beautiful thing I ever saw.

All my What If…has been erased.

8 January 2012
I have just spent the afternoon with my beautiful seven-year-old friend Lainey. She told me that she had seen something on a film that was so scary that she couldn't even bring herself to talk about it. She said she thought about it all the time. She looked genuinely concerned. She then very seriously asked me, 'If I worry about something will it happen?'

The very obvious answer to this question, is of course... No. Hell no. Or the more child friendly, Heck no.

But it made me think... How often do we adults entertain 'scary thoughts' and allow them to run rampant in our minds until we feel scared, insecure and upset? How often do we worry about events that have never happened, probably will never happen? And yet our fear is as genuine as whatever ghoul or monster my seven-year-old little friend had envisioned.

I explained to Lainey that fear was often not real, nor was it based on anything true to life. I asked her, if her worry or her thoughts had made things come true in the past? She admitted that this had not happened. I explained that the film she had watched was fake, and that even if we thought really hard about the scary thing, it would never, ever happen. And then we stood there in the kitchen, mid brownie making session, and we thought about something scary and we waited to see if it happened, and of course, it didn't.

A big toothy smile broke out on her face, and I hope, that perhaps she learned something at an early age that she might take with her in the future. I know I did. And I know that next time I catch myself imagining my life going terribly wrong, based upon a generally fictional thought pattern. I'll stop, I'll think of Lainey and her horrible scary film, and I'll smile because no, worry does not make things happen. And so, it's very simple, we can recognize this and we choose to stop worrying. Easier said than done? Well if a seven year old can do it, I think perhaps I can too. Monsters don't exist you know!

My body is playing me up. I can't do what I could a few months ago. And it sucks. It sucks so bad. Because I know now that I took my healthy, youthful, flexible body for granted. I took it for granted that I could bend over without getting out of breath. I took it for granted that a twenty-minute session in the gym would not induce mind-bending tiredness. I lived in my body, but did I really appreciate it? Did I love it? Or did I spend time trying to make it bend to my will and behave?

Like a naughty child, my body seemed rebellious. But the thing is, it wasn't, it was doing what I needed all along. It was giving me a shell, a home, a place to exist and experience life from. It was me. It was inseparable from me. I owe it a lot of love, because it is the only thing I will ever truly know. My body was not rebellious, but my mind was. My mind was too quick to judge, too quick to compare my love handles to that of some starlet plastered across the cover of a perfume advert. We should switch the focus from our bodies to our minds and in doing so we may find that self-love is easier to come by than we think.

Happily I am only pregnant and my fitness and my usual body will return. And when it does I will never again take my beloved body for granted. I will pledge to honor my fitness, my ability to move, my alertness every single day. I will honor it in making nourishing food choices and keeping the movement well oiled and strong with exercise, eating healthy and running around after my new baba! I will honor it with a mental appreciation too. I won't allow those negativities to sink in, the ones that say because I am not of glamour girl proportions, I am not worthy.

We are all worthy. All our bodies are perfect in their imperfections. As long as they play house to our hearts and souls, they are utterly perfect. Vanity is but a whisper in the breeze and it is one that we should allow to bypass us.

I will from now on conclude that I love my body, it is a temple, irrespective of whether or not that temple is an old mud shack or one fitted out with full on six pack style altar. There is, as we all know...no place like home.

9 January 2012

Woke up feeling massively anxious and borderline angry. I was quietly simmering and seething for no obvious reason. I had to bite my tongue to avoid unnecessary confrontation with James, who had done nothing wrong. He had, however, slept through his alarm and missed his lift to work. This meant I had to take him to work at an ungodly early hour. Rather than be a bitch about it I grinned and made him breakfast. Secretly I really, really wanted to be a bitch about it. Instead I pleasantly drove him to work smiling all the way, grimacing internally.

I couldn't help but notice a massive and stunning full moon. Perhaps this is having some effect on me? I am werewolf woman, the waters of my womb pulled to the dark-side. Who knows, since the sun came up fully I'm feeling lighter and less angry. Perhaps Mother Luna was tugging a little too strong on my front heavy centre of gravity causing my pleasant tides to turn.

How wonderful, a lovely lady named Annie read a blog I wrote about pregnancy grumps and is kindly sending me a copy of pregnancy meditations CD, *Healthy Pregnancy in a Box.* What a lovely gift. Maybe that moon has shifted and made the tides turn for the better. And maybe all things happen for a reason and I got the grumps just so I'd really appreciate this lovely present.

In spite of that it seems I can't win today. Now I've discovered that my favorite pregnancy 'go to' drink on a night out is horrible for fetal development. Oh good lord what is a girl to do? This drink has been my occasional non-alcoholic naughty treat, but now I'm told I could be damaging my Poppyseed. I've read so much on having a baby, but aside from having a library downloaded into my head, I'm not sure what more I can do.

I feel like a really bad mum now. I should be reading more, I should be doing more, I should be buying pure, organic food and shunning anything other than the best of the best of everything. I can't keep up with it all. I feel like such a failure. I'm too busy with all my own various workings and maybe I'm overlooking what's important. Does everyone feel like this? Christ ,I'm not even wearing deodorant for fear of damaging the baby, I stink. I stopped wearing nail varnish for the whole first trimester and walked around with vile two inch long roots for the fear of bleach, but I've been happily guzzling the aforementioned drink like it's going out of fashion, well maybe once or twice a week. What a total mega fail disaster.

Okay I've calmed down. Following some frantic texting back and forth, James called me up and said all the right things. It's like he has memorized some kind of 'placating pregnant women' script. It's amazing, and it works, and I love him so much for saying all the nice things and staying calm whilst I'm being tearful and hysterical.

Hopefully my red puffy face will relax a little by the time he is here. He is being such a trooper. Whatever he has learnt, or read, or decided, is like magic. I feel much better now.

I think all this moodiness started last night when I made Carbonara and went to taste it and realized it had meat in it. I'm a veggie and I had to whip something up real quick for me and try to forget I'd just accidentally ingested pig. That put me on edge and the fall out has been spectacular.

Molly cat is now doing her best to calm me down with some Kitty love. My family is colluding to make me see sense. Love them all to death!

Jan 11th 2012

Today was our second hospital baby scan (and goddess willing) the last.

Today for the first time ever we saw our little girl's heart beating. On the other scans this eluded us. It looked like a little jumping coffee bean or a tulip. Opening and closing. Opening and closing. Pumping life into her, deep inside me. All was healthy and well with aortas and ventricles in the right place, doing what they should. And of course, so much more than just biology. But I don't have the words. So this will do.

That was today's miracle, my baby girl's heart, nothing more, and nothing less. Perfect. Amen.

11 January 2012 ctd…

A little more info… It was the full scan of baby today. All was well with Poppyseed. James didn't realize quite how important today's scan was and I didn't enlighten him. I figured he is more of a worrier than he admits. The last scan saw him deathly silent until we saw the heartbeat, and so I decided that it was best that one of us is oblivious to the full facts. I did mention to him on the way to hospital that this was the full scan. He didn't ask what that meant. I figure that sometimes ignorance is bliss. I needed him to be strong and chatty for me, so why rock the boat? I was vaguely nervous, but in my heart I knew all would be well. We had a student doing the scan, and as such he was overly thorough. Which meant Poppyseed was super examined, every last bit of her. It was a little intimidating as they moved from one body part or organ to the next. Happily, her parts are in perfect order and yes, we double-checked, she is still a girl!

You may remember when we went for the first scan and bumped into a friend Kim, that we hitherto had not known was pregnant. She was there again and looking far happier than the first time. So lovely to chat to her and compare notes. Such a strong, independent soul she is, I'm very lucky to have James about to do 'man' stuff. Her husband is working away for at least the next five weeks and so she is going it alone; which she handles with considerable panache. What a fantastic independent example she will be to her little baby. I like to think I'm independent, but in comparison I'm really not and I find the quality very admirable. I shall have to work on that one.

She told me that she had recently dreamed about me, that I had a big pregnant belly. Which I can envisage coming true in the next few months, alongside her own!

Speaking of dreams... Last night I dreamt I had had Poppyseed and she was a grown woman, a very glamorous, beautiful and tall woman. This didn't faze me one bit. I went in to look after her and she asked me to change her nappy and explained to me how I would do it. We trotted off to the bathroom and unbothered I set about the task. I guess this dream reflects my life from now on. Once that girl is here I'll be happily helping her clear up her shit for the rest of her life. A task I am clearly more than contented to do.

In the dream someone else had pooped in the bidet. This frustrated me no end, yet I was happy to sort out this adult woman's nappy. A sign that she alone will hold a place in my heart as the only person whose mess I will be content to deal with!

15 January 2012

Thinking of Grace as a middle name for Poppyseed. And Faith. Also toyed with Elizabeth or maybe Rebecca after my Mum. Her first name was easy to come by. We had decided it years ago before we even wanted children. It is James's Grandma's name. He loved that Grandma dearly and she passed away soon after I met him. I met her once at a party and she spoke to me, it was loud and I had to ask her to repeat herself. In the end we gave up. I never will know what she said to me. Probably something boring like 'nice to meet you', but who knows…

We have spent a wonderful country weekend in Yorkshire with friends Gary and Gaynor and their little daughter, Anais. Gary and James can have a drink and celebrate their birthdays together. Gaynor and I can talk babies, as we are both pregnant. It was fabulous to be with people – eat, drink (soft drinks) and be merry. Great to have so many of us yelling at trash TV so loudly that I lost the plot of the show. I felt drunk, but I promise I absolutely wasn't. Maybe drunk on fresh air and good friends! It was lovely to have little Anais around being charming and cute and an ideal future role model to my unborn!

Walked a lot to and from the famous village of Haworth. At one point, I had an incredible shooting pain in my buttock. It lasted for a split second and hurt like nothing I've felt before, but it passed quickly and came to nothing. I think my body may be starting a rebellion.

I was rather impressed by mine and Gaynor's willingness to hike through freezing cold fields, dodging patches of ice and trying not to stumble over the rocks and heather of the wild Yorkshire moors. It was all very *Wuthering Heights*, but with Kathy being knocked up and Heathcliff being far more comical.

All that walking has given me a bruised feeling coccyx. It feels peculiar but is hardly disabling. I shan't let it slow me down too much.

Gaynor is a month or so ahead of me with her pregnancy. Her baby was moving a lot. She was often grabbing someone's hand to feel the little one squirming around. I still get the occasional kick, but they are hard to catch for someone else to feel them. I'm excited to get to her stage so that James can feel his little girl more often and more definitively.

Have finally caved and bought some maternity clothes. Before pregnancy, I threw all my leggings away in a fit of classy dressing. I now own a pair of pregnancy leggings and may I say they are truly brilliant. Classy or otherwise they are so damned comfy, and that's all that matters right now.

I'm feeling determined to focus now on me and baby. I want to buy a special baby rattle. Rattles are very important to Shamanic healers, and my girl is a little natural Shaman in the making. This will be a gift for my baby's soul. If she chooses not to be a Shaman, then she can at least give it a good shake and a chew.

17 January 2012

Finally I have started to really read *Hypnobirthing* by Marie Mongan. Only a few chapters into my book, and I'm already feeling empowered, inspired and even excited to give birth. The philosophy really resonates with me. It states that pain in birth stems from fear. The fact birth has been made medical and stigmatized as a traumatic event adds up to one big fear factor. According to Hypnobirthing, labor should not naturally be painful or something to be afraid of. Apparently, many other cultures don't find it painful and nor do other animals because neither have a fear of birth. I love this idea. I'm going to go with it. I want my birth to be as natural and stress free as possible. I want Poppyseed's entry into this life to reflect peace, grace and love, not screaming, fear or medical intrusion. I'll see how it goes. I've signed James and I up for a course with a Hypnobirthing Doula, Mia Scotland, who has a great reputation as a birthing expert. Strangely, I can't wait.

Momma's been doing her thinking again... I wish sometimes I were born as an Amazonian Rainforester or some such similar existence. I wish that ambition would drift out of my head and let me be. I desire a life that is uncomplicated and simple, and yet day in day out I stuff my brain with thought toxins and ram my diary full to bursting. The thing is, I have been at this spiritual lark for a good few years now, and my brain is far less full than it used to be, and since getting knocked up, my diary too is emptying rapidly. Yet still, like many a good human before me, I fail to let it be, relax, chill, release and all that other good stuff.

But this is important. Releasing our lives to the universe, to the goddess almighty or to whatever powers you believe in is vital to living a soulful life. We simply must give up the controlling aspects of existence that see us clamoring for a particular ending, a specific finale to our train of thoughts. Our thoughts will rarely create the existence we think that they will. I believe that you cannot concentrate on an exact outcome and receive it. Well you can, but in rigidly controlling what you receive through exacting thoughts, you may not get what you actually need. I believe it's better to hold a hope, have faith in it and then accept what you are given. In accepting what you are given you trust that this gift is the right thing for you. No matter how much it isn't what you thought it would be, it is right for you here and now.

We can practice release every single moment. Whenever your brain starts to toddle off down lanes of fantasy, then you simply have to stop that track of thinking. There is no point hiking up and down the paths of imagination when reality is a whole different color. So instead, don't entertain it. Relax, release, and chill. Let it be.

That said, fantasies are where great dreams start, fantasies are what changes life. So in our mindfulness, we must know which fantasies to entertain and which to dump in the wilderness. Only we can know that, and only when the time is right can certain dreams be dropped and others begun.

So all I am saying, whilst good and relevant, is pointless anyway. A girl's got to dream…

18 January 2012

Thinking about cash today. I'm not a math person, far from it, so numbers, money and sums are largely avoided in the general hemisphere of my brain. My finances, or rather our finances, are totally empty due to the repaid car loan and it's only with a small loan from James's mum, Beverley that we continue with the plans for the house and Poppyseed's room.

I'm also refocusing my attention on what I really love. I've dropped my meditation class and my tarot reading. Apart from the day job, these things did bring in extra cash, but at the expense of my sanity, so I've cleared some space financially and mentally and I'm waiting for things to fill it. I've been asked to blog for three different sites, entirely unpaid, but it's all good writing practice and publicity for my work. One of these opportunities is for a big American TV show's website. I definitely can't complain, I still have the old reliable day job, but as I am working from home now, things could not be more perfect.

Money is so overrated. I'm glad to have some, and happy it pays for my life, as I know it. More important right now, is time. Time to be with James, time for baby belly and time to write. Time spent happily is the greatest currency.

20 January 2012

My belly is really popping out now. Before it looked the same, but bigger, now it looks all round and distended. My belly button appears different too and I only assume it is working its way inside out. I'm so glad to be looking pregnant though, it's a relief. It is far preferable, vanity speaking, to looking portly.

I am now enduring horrid shooting pains much like the one I endured in Yorkshire. They stem from my coccyx, down my left buttock. They only last a few seconds, but they are sharp and horrific. Making me catch my breath and wince. They have also, thus far, put paid to my gym visits. I did attend once with hopes of 'working' the pain out and loosening it up; that didn't work and in fact made it worse. I guess I'll see how it goes and swimming may be a good option now. According to my pregnancy resources it's all quite normal and I should stay active. Though I should also avoid putting pressure on the area. Which is impossible, the area endures pressure no matter what I do, or don't do. It's just 'one of those' areas, essential for all movement.

Maybe the cosmos is trying to slow me down. Good Luck with that. I'm pregnant and not disabled and this girl cannot become a couch potato – I just can't… Or can I?

Breaking news: I've just done some research and found that my belly is now sticking out a little further than my boobs. Which, given the size of them is a remarkable achievement. I am now officially, undeniably pregnant.

22 January 2912

Had a shocking experience yesterday. I'd spent a lovely day with my best friend Roisin and driving home, I had a nasty occurrence. Wheeling my way through the countryside I saw a car behind pull out to overtake me. Frighteningly, I could see a line of cars coming around the corner up ahead. I could also judge by speed and distance that there was a high likelihood of impact round about when the oncoming and overtaking car were right next to me. Panicking, I didn't know whether to brake and enable the overtaking car to get round quicker, or speed up so he could slot in behind me. In all honesty, I think I did a bit of both. My mind went blank and it seemed that a head on collision was inevitable. The only thing that went through my mind was, of course, that I might never meet Poppyseed.

Somehow, both cars appeared to pass me at the same time, without hitting each other. I pretty much cried all the way home. I felt like I'd experienced an 'almost' near death experience. One that amounted to nothing but had time been a second or so different, could have been devastating. I got home as quickly as I could and had a good cry on James's shoulder.

I don't want to make more of this non-event than necessary, but it has had a profound effect. Firstly, I felt my first bang of maternal protectiveness and secondly, I felt so incredibly grateful to still be here. As a result, I can think of nothing more than looking after my baby, making her safe, welcome and hoping that we all live happy, healthy, long lives. All we have is the moment. So, in this moment, I'm off to lie down and rub my belly for a while.

25 January 2012
It's been a dark week. It was Ellen's funeral yesterday, which was exhausting. I felt somewhat out of place there; I didn't know Ellen hugely well. She used to be my boss and she was great mates with my best friend. I saw her a couple of times socially, she was always the life and soul, cheeky, charming and terribly behaved – in a good way. So many people turned up at the funeral, so many friends. It was a hardcore catholic service, terribly impersonal and perhaps a little on the staid and judgmental side. I guess that is what the family wanted. The end was very moving when the priests stood down and the family spoke about Ellen. That was deeply moving. She was a much-loved Woman. She will be missed.

After a tiring day I also learned that James has been asked to do a gig in Spain in a week. I reacted so badly to this. A mix of tiredness, hunger, exhaustion, pregnancy and just plain old paranoia settled heavy on my brain. James and I have spent a year getting over the horridness that happened in tandem with band and music related stuff at the end of 2010. 2011 was hugely healing and restorative and we are in a better place than ever. Yet I let my tiredness get the better of me, and I panicked. Panicked that his very cool trip to Spain could, somehow, spell disaster for him and me. Is this a woman thing? I have friends whose heads swing the same way with similar news. Is it an insecurity thing, or a pregnant, tired can't-think-straight thing?

I know that if I told James I was going to Spain in a week, he'd be nothing but supportive. Anyway I went a 'bit weird', then I sucked it up, had a word with myself and I'm now feeling more myself and happy for him. I guess no matter how much you have faith in a person, or in your life, occasionally negative thinking floors you. I'm not proud of it, but I'm a work in progress. After a good night's sleep I feel fine, content, relaxed. Thank Goddess it's now, rather than when I'm heavily pregnant and he may have had to turn it down. That would have been worse. After a year working on the house, on himself and on putting me first, an all expenses paid trip to Spain is much deserved.

Baby has been kicking loads. James has felt a few more now. Last night she really did boot him in the hand. It's all so real. As are the painful shooting pains I still get down the back of my left hip. I'm keeping up some gentle exercise and determined to carry on being me until such time as Miss Poppyseed has her way.

25 January 2012
Just looking online at flights to go to the USA later in the year to visit family. Had to search for two adults and one child. My, oh my. What a strange and cool experience. Most unusual!

25 January 2012
Went out for dinner last night with James at about 5.30pm. It was bog standard decent pub grub. I was pretty full afterwards but thought nothing of it. By 9pm I was exhausted and still feeling so full of food, but it had been an early start and I needed bed. Woke up at 10.30pm after a couple of hours sleep and felt as though I had still only just eaten. The food from five hours previously seemed to be sat on my lungs, never mind reached my stomach yet. My cat Molly came and lay on my chest as she often does, and I found I just couldn't breathe. It was an absolutely horrendous feeling. So the rebellion has begun. Miss P is having her way. Minute portions and plenty of them is the way forward!

27 January 2012
Well what a week! Near (almost) death experiences, funerals and then I win an award for *The High Heeled Guide to Spiritual Living*. Interest in my books seems to be upping a little. I did request in my letter to the universe for that to happen. Normally my letters are vague, but I decided to be specific and it's seemingly paying off. I won the *Prediction Magazine Best Book Award*. I, of course, made a specific request for a healthy, happy baby and family too – and so far so good. Come to think of it, I made a vision board many months ago, before I was pregnant requesting these specific things too. I wanted to be pregnant; I wanted my books to do well. Wishes granted. Thank you cosmos.

This morning I dropped James off at his friends so he can get a lift to work, and I went back to bed. Poppyseed started to kick. So every time she kicked, I squeezed my tummy muscles to give her a hug. She responded. She kicked more than ever. It was beautiful. In the end I simply had to roll over and get some sleep, but it was so precious to play and connect with my now rather large Poppyseed.

I am conscious that baby can now hear things, so I am trying to keep things interesting. I just downloaded music from my childhood, Bruce Springsteen and Meatloaf. So far she hasn't kicked any objections. Previous to this US Rock-fest we spent the morning with nature-based meditation music on, so hopefully I'm striking a good balance. Is it music that is the food of love? Well the only love I can give her is tummy clenches, pokes and sound, so hopefully I'll be thrilling her senses. Play on.

29 January 2012
This coming Wednesday I will be six months pregnant – twenty-four weeks. The past few days have seen me change in my thinking. My focus is less on me and my pregnancy and more on

the coming child. Was even considering what outfit to get Poppyseed for a friend's wedding just after her birth. Today I was looking at nursery paint and prams and hugely enjoying it. I'm feeling really excited and my learning about hypnobirthing has taken the fear out of birth. Reading more and more about the theory of hypnobirthing has left me with so much excitement and happiness. I've gone from abject terror, to a real desire to get busy birthing and to enjoy it. I intend to absolutely expect the best, best birth, the best baby, the best conversion to motherhood and why not? Negative expectations create a dire reality. I truly believe that thinking wholesomely will forge and create a better future. Hypnobirthing has made the lead up to birth bearable because I'm no longer afraid of pain or trauma that I previously associated with birth.

Poppyseed has been moving around more and more. If she is still for too long I miss her and give her a little poke! It's a heart-warming feeling to know she is in there chilling out and progressing. I so can't wait to meet her.

I did a radio interview today talking about my books. It turns out that the host runs spiritual baby workshops worldwide, working on in-utero baby communication. I love a happy non-coincidence and so listened carefully to her advice. She advised me not to cut the 'cord' for at least an hour after birth, as this interrupts baby's connection with babies home, babies source, me. I like this theory a lot. James is not so keen but willing to forego his reservations to entertain my hippy ways.

Speaking of James, he too seems to be suffering crazy dreams. I guess it's not all hormonal, it's life and it's a big deal, which does not go unnoticed by the subconscious. So together we lay at night in adventurous dream realms slowly coming to terms with the adventure ahead.

31 January 2012

I have woken up feeling full of motivational patter. I have already told James that we are not given anything in this life that we can't handle, but it's only when we show weakness that things get difficult. I then imparted some wisdom to my cat – there's nothing to fear except fear itself. I also had a word with Poppyseed, patting my tummy, growling and saying 'I'm ready baby, bring it on.'

Yes, I know, all very bizarre, I can't even blame this surge of self-help guru behavior on too much coffee as I am abstaining from my morning cuppa.

James asked last night (jokingly) if I was sure I was pregnant. Other than the protruding bump, I'm 6 months gone with relatively little to show for it. I'm so proud of that. I've had aches and pains but I carried on regardless and feel better for it. I've eaten well, but not gone mad. I've exercised nicely but not gone mad. I feel full of the joys of spring, super positive and determined to allow pregnancy to be an incredible gift, not an affliction. Hence, perhaps, my super motivation side making itself known today. I'm cheerleading, rousing the troops, getting ready for taking no nonsense and being a loving, badass momma.

Rise and shine sleepyheads, the day is dawning and the day is ours for the taking!

So why do some people treat pregnancy as an affliction? I guess for many it really, truly is... But my pregnancy is going great, it is empowering me. I've never felt more myself than when I have been growing a new person.

1 February 2012

Well yesterday's upbeat attitude did not last. Around about lunchtime I went into an utter decline and ended the day feeling quite low. I think I peaked far too soon. Although this change of mood was brought about in part by the rabbit wars occurring in my garden...

We have three rabbits, George, Maggie May and Lady Madonna, Lady M and Maggie M have been fighting; they are sisters, but need neutering and I've been horribly lax about it. The fighting yesterday was awful. I felt such a failure and in turn James started encouraging me to give the rabbits to a shelter. But if I can't manage sweet little fluffy bunnies, where will I stand on a sentient human child? Feeling weak, vulnerable and sorry for myself, I agreed to the shelter idea. I then spent quite some time crying about it (what hormones?). Sleep didn't help. Meditation didn't help.

Well that was yesterday and thankfully today, I feel different (again).

I have realized that I've not helped this fighting situation one bit. I've been a bad rabbit momma.

Giving them up to a shelter breaks my heart; it makes me feel a failure, like I'm caving in to pressure and stress. The thing is, I work from home, and I have the time to do what I need to do for them. I just need to do it. So today I'm making momma rabbit efforts. It was easy. I know James isn't happy, but I hope he can try to trust me on this one. And yes there may well be some time when I struggle with them, but I may struggle with everything for a little while. I'm not ready to give up the image of me breast-feeding this summer in the garden with my snuffle-buns bouncing around.

Mother Earth does not give up. So I'm rolling up my sleeves and getting on with the job. This is a turning point and I and the rabbits are going to be happy damn it. If indeed I ever do give them away, it will not be to a shelter. It will be to happy homes. If that happens, the homes will find us...if it is meant to be?

As I was petting Maggie May, I noticed a bit of crumpled newspaper in her cage. I was compelled to pick it up. It said 'snub Maggie' on it. It was a real '*Charlotte's Web*' moment. I gave her a really big cuddle and let her out for some bun bun fun. The newspaper tearing Goddess has spoken and who am I not to abide?

2 February 2012
Last night I dreamt I should weigh myself. I dreamt that I would have put on about a stone. I've been avoiding weighing myself, but as the dream made me feel so positive about it I literally dusted off the scales and got on. I was pleased to see I have put on one stone exactly (that's the first time I ever expressed pleasure at putting on weight!) During pregnancy a gal is supposed (by law) to put on 2 stones. So six months in, with four left to go I'm really happy with that. I feel strangely proud of myself. It's important I keep 'me' during this pregnancy, as I don't need the extra burden of having to re-find 'me' when the baby is here. So I'm very happy and thankful for that psychic dream. Let's be honest, a stone is easily accountable for, a bit of belly, a bit of baby, a bit of fat around my hips, placenta, extra blood, lots of new boob! In fact I think most of that weight is new boob. From a DD, I must be bordering on a G cup round about now – Lucky James.

3 February 2012
I dreamt vividly last night that I gave birth. It was entirely painless and no injury was caused. Hopefully this is a true indicator of the future. This morning the thought of having a pizza tonight was the only thing that got me out of bed.

I enjoyed a mid-morning emotional meltdown on a video call to my Mum and her partner Karen today. I misinterpreted something Momma did (shook her head, or sighed or something inane) and I presumed she vastly disapproved of my life. I went away and wound myself up about it, then rang her up in floods of tears to tell her how happy I am and how she shouldn't worry or disapprove of anything.

I'm very conscious of the fact that Mum was there for me when I had a difficult start to 2011, she saw the chaos firsthand and witnessed her little girl hanging by a thread. Since then, I've made choices with a creeping feeling that she wishes I did something else.

Whether I overreacted or not, it cleared the air and I feel better. Everyone loves everyone and I am left pretty exhausted by my outburst. Though it was an outburst worth having, it paves the way for a nice future with no one (me) second-guessing what others might be thinking.

5 February 2012

James is in Marbella and I'm snowed in. Though I miss James, it's been nice just to do my own things without interruption. Yesterday I went to see Rosh and randomly ended up doing a workout DVD in the living room. Poor Rosh nearly keeled over with exhaustion whilst pregnant old me held her own and got through the whole thing with only a few adaptations. As soon as snow started to fall, I headed home, picked up some delicious healthy dinner, locked all the doors and got cozy. Today, I've played in the snow with the cats and rabbits, done my homework for my course, done my pregnancy yoga DVD and am now planning a nice bath and a night in front of the TV.

James will be back home early tomorrow and I have a busy week ahead so chilling out this weekend has been a godsend. I do miss him though. It can be hard to be the one stuck at home whilst the other is off gallivanting. I know if I were off gallivanting, James would be fine, barely miss me at all. I wonder sometimes if that is the difference between men and women? Us gals, seem, in my experience, to have a deeper need to be with their other halves? Maybe it's a nesting thing, or a homemaker gene? Maybe it's a sociological thing and I'm suffering under the belief I should be the all suffering, ever-waiting wifey! Who knows? But one thing is sure, I am looking forward to his return, I'm waiting for it. I'm doing fine, but if I'm really honest with myself I am waiting…

I have felt particularly tired and blurry-minded in the past few days so being stuck indoors because of the snow is welcome. I am a little bit of a danger to myself; I'm constantly knocking things over and breaking stuff. The toll of which has meant that despite buying new drinks glasses recently, we are perilously low again. My blender has had its day too as I managed to smash that too. Most concerning was leaving the house yesterday. I nearly fell sideways over the welcome mat, and, on arriving at Rosh's I put the handbrake on insufficiently causing the car to roll down a hill with me half in and half out of it. Caffeine may not be ideal for a baby but right now it is essential to me, it's a rough compromise but a couple of cups of tea may well save my life and limb!

I have been thinking about how often I've said in this diary that I don't want to change and I want to keep being me. I think perhaps these are throwaway comments as I certainly am changing. I'm not the same gal I was six months ago, and in four month's time, I'll be different still, and that's okay, I embrace it. I hope to grow with pregnancy and motherhood. Things will be different. Some things I'm sure will remain the same.

There is much focus in society on how much parenthood can change a person and how it can make life harder, but we live in a very selfish society that sometimes sees kids as obligations or accessories rather than a path to something greater and more meaningful. Parenthood is viewed as a problem to solve, a risk, something that must be handled or else parents may lose their selves and their sanity. I guess that is why I've partially bought into the 'keeping me' mantra, but, for the record, none of us 'keep me'. Life has its ways of ensuring that 'me' is always fluid, changing and moveable. Kids or no kids, there is no such thing as a tangible 'me'. There is only the moment. I want every moment with baby to be one spent in love, learning and growth. I want to follow my instinct and forget anything I ever read so I can work it out as a unique entity in this beautiful harmony of big and little soul. I don't need to keep 'me'. What I need is only an appreciation of the moment, every last one of them!

Just been playing with Poppyseed. Decided to have a lie down on the bed. Jimi cat came and lay on top of me, sprawled right up my torso. I placed my hands lightly on my belly and waited for the kicks to come. Spent some time deep breathing and sending positive, happy thoughts down to Miss P. Even spoke to her and let her know what a nice life and birth we would have. Whenever she kicked, which was often, I'd squeeze my belly in to hug her. This went on for ten minutes with Jimi perched atop all the action quite happily. I made a concerted effort to imagine beautiful, healing rainbow colors flowing through my breath, down my arms and into my little girl. I hope she loved it. I adore these quiet moments of connection.

6 February 2012
I'm so tired. I feel it in my head and eyes mostly. I'm sleeping fine though, other than the four or five trips to the toilet every night. Working from home means lots less stress, so I think I can wholly put this tiredness down to pregnancy. I was going to go to the gym this morning, but it's so cold and snowy. I can always go later, or do one of my pregnancy DVDs. James is back today. I

expect he'll be tired too, possibly significantly hungover also.

Oh god, the tiredness has progressed into a massive mood swing. Just found myself sobbing into a tissue because I'm not sat on a hot and gorgeous beach. Feeling utterly sorry for myself. I know I'm being ridiculous and people are being sweet to me, but I just really wish I could get whisked off to a stunning sunny beach somewhere. I just want to lay there, no work, no books to write, and no animals to worry about. I need some time and some space, headspace more than anything. I need some space to breathe. I need to have some time outside of my routine, outside of everything. I'd really just like to feel warm. God I'm tired.

7 February 2012

My exhaustion was not helpful. Poor James thought I was being weird with him on his return; maybe I was, a little. Maybe I missed him more than I let on… Having had a great weekend my moodiness didn't cap it off too well for either of us. Needless to say I feel horrible about it; I'm not very pleased with myself, but at the same time I'm in total sympathy with myself. I am somewhat out of control of how tired I feel, but I wish I'd had a few minutes to centre myself before James got home. I was so excited to see him, but it was all washed down the drain by my out of character behavior. I'm not even sure what I did, I just wasn't myself. I should have greeted him with a big hug and smile. But instead I wanted him to see how tired and needy I was. So that characterized the greeting. I guess I was attention seeking. But it was bad timing. He thought I was not happy to see him. I really was though!

Don't you just love it when you mess up and you know you should have known better? That's how I feel, so frustrated with myself.

Whilst I believe there are no mistakes, there certainly are such things as freaking hormones, which can lead to lapses. More than anything I detest hurting people's feelings and I think that's what I've done, I made my lovely fella feel shitty about being home when he was so looking forward to being here and chilling. I feel I'm cracking up; not good. Only a few days ago I was on top of the world and happy. Pregnancy rocks, but this aspect of it is a rock around my neck. I won't miss it.

8 February 2012
Hopefully I'm back to normal today. Went to the theatre last night with Mum and Karen and saw a funny female comedy duo, Lip Service. It was lovely to put on a dress and get out of the house for something other than the gym. Indeed it gave me a whole new perspective on the bump. It's pretty huge. I nearly fell over several times because my eyes were firmly posted on my own belly. It seemed to be leading the way everywhere; it was hard not to stare downward.

Today I am twenty-five weeks. Which gives me fifteen to spare. This latest batch of moodiness has been a bummer, but let's hope that's all done with for now.

James and I are slightly perturbed by the math. Fifteen weeks. Whilst we still have over a third of the pregnancy left it's all feeling very real today. Discussions started of massive clear outs, massive, ruthless clear outs. Indeed James decided to test my metal by querying the staying power of some of our potted plants. I decided it wasn't worth the row and on a whim threw a load of things out (half dead plants not included). Some of the stuff I binned, it turns out, was stuff that James had rather I hadn't thrown, but I guess ruthlessness has its price.

I went for lunch with friends today, I tried to cross my legs under the table and couldn't do it, which was a first. I also feel like I'm starting to waddle. As well as waddling I'm clumsy with my body, high heels are still most definitely out. I'm sure those celebrities 'papped' wearing six inch heels must only have a few yards to go, before, away from the cameras, they slip out of their Laboutins and into their smelly old reliable sneakers. High heels hurt my back and as I have no-one papping me, it's flats all the way.

9 February 2012

Today started off with a fascinating event, I dropped James off in the morning and was headed up the dual carriageway home. Up ahead I could see police lights and what appeared to be a whole bunch of people in the road. It was about 4.15am and so this was unexpected. I simply presumed someone had been run over or there was some kind of incident cracking off. I slowed down as I got closer and my mouth fell open in astonishment as the 'people' moved across into the other lane and continued to trot the wrong way down past me. The 'people' were five brown and white horses, presumably escaped from the nearby fields. They looked happy enough with their police escort and didn't startle at my presence either.

As a keen animal lover and believer in all things having spiritual meaning, I am yet to decipher this. Whatever message those beautiful creatures had for me is probably only as relevant as the big smile they placed on my face.

Today also turned out to be my first pregnant stranger interaction. Thus far I've hidden my small bump from prying eyes but today, in my haste to grab milk and toilet roll, I had my coat unbuttoned and was told by the lady at the counter that if she'd realized my condition she would have assisted me. Baby bump is most definitely visible and I couldn't help but fulfill my glowing mother-to-be role and answer all the nice lady's questions about when I was due. She did kindly tell me I should slow down, and perhaps I agree. Needless to say, the shopping I intended to buy expanded once in-store and carrying three heavy bags left me a little breathless. I haven't done any exercise since Sunday and I do intend to scale it back a bit, but I'm not yet ready to succumb to the chorus of panic about my exercising. Not quite yet.

I finally had an antenatal appointment today. Nothing to report except that I heard Miss P's heartbeat, which made me smile so big and wide. Love that little girl!

Tonight I have been waddling around rubbing my belly and eating spoonfuls of honey. This pregnancy bliss was interrupted briefly by walking into the cat scratching post and stubbing my toe – twice. I sounded like a cat on heat with the screeches I let out.

I have been reading my copies of *The Mother* a great alternative-parenting magazine. This made me feel all goddess like and maternal – hence the belly rubbing and honey eating. I would feel better if I'd harvested the honey locally or even better garnered it from a hive at the bottom of my garden, but I didn't, it came from the local European supermarket, cheap as chips. I must try harder. I will visit my local farm store as soon as possible to purchase some honey from the bums of local bees. This playing at being mother earth is hard work and I'll never get it as finely tuned as some of the women in *The Mother*. But my heart is in the right place and I'm aware, this is a good enough start; followed, of course, by local honey. For this moment a mix of EU and Non EU hives will simply have to do.

✡

11 February 2012

It's been an intense weekend. I've had some real, vivid, wacky dreams, chock full of celebrities and zany story lines. Madonna was there and comedian Lenny Henry was my boyfriend. And that's just the bits that I remember.

I also think I have received more compliments this weekend than I have altogether in the past few years. I'm now fully informed that pregnancy suits me. Which is lovely, I can live with that, much thanks to the many women who have rallied forward with kind comments on my appearance and choice of pregnancy attire. It really has meant a lot, especially as I've felt like a front heavy waddling duck of late!

Out beyond the crazy dreams and compliments, I have undergone something very powerful. I've been on my therapy course all weekend. This week during our therapy practice I chose to address guilt. Guilt is one of those things that has popped up time and time again in my life. I sometimes feel as if I'm responsible for everyone else's happiness, or lack thereof, so I feel guilty if I can't make them happy, or they are unhappy irrespective of whatever I do.

I think that this occasionally has led to me being overly concerned with my actions and their repercussions. I tend to apologize a lot, sometimes I think, too much, and unnecessarily. It's also perhaps contributed to a secret inner dialogue with myself that has a habit of popping up in times of stress and conflicts. We all have a 'secret inner life', but I can see where mine has been damaging at times, and compounded with guilt has made me less of the person I could be. I feel that sometimes, unless we have done something really bad, we need to take guilt and shove it.

I often hear of 'mothers guilt' and it seems to be a fairly acknowledged phenomena. I know my mum certainly feels 'mother's guilt', always wondering what she did wrong when we were children, how might she have been better. I admit I get frustrated with her over this. I come from a place where I believe all things happen for a reason and so any 'mistakes' she felt she made, were needed by us on a deep soul level. Life is never smooth, people are not perfect, and my brothers and I are doing more than fine. She must drop this terrible self-torturing guilt.

But she doesn't, she carries on feeling it. I guess she can't help it. I guess so many momma's do.

To me it's a wasted emotion. No-one can change the past; they shouldn't either even if they could. I think my Mum was very brave in the past. I admire her. I admire myself, I don't want to be any different. And if she changed the past then she is meddling with who I am. I don't like that.

So I dealt with my guilt via our therapeutic practice, a little hypnosis, and a little shamanic magic. I don't want to be feeling guilt for anything I do with Poppyseed. I'll do my absolute best, I'm sure I'll make mistakes, we all do. But no regrets, no guilt. Guilt doesn't solve anything. Love free from guilt or conditions solves alot. Maybe I'm being naïve but my mistakes I intend to salve with love.

15 February 2012

The dreams just keep coming, always chock a block, full of celebrities. Last night Madonna and her daughter, Lourdes featured heavily, but I can't remember why. The main thrust of the dream was that I was giving marital advice to Russell Brand relating to his divorce to songstress Katy Perry. Most unusually Russell and I conducted most of our 'therapy' fully dressed in the bath.

So the only question left is which superstars will grace my dreams tonight? Miss P is clearly attracting them all in. I ought to rent space in my head to the paparazzi.

After spending the weekend sat down on my course I've been like an achy and creaky old woman. I've done some exercise gym/Pilates/shopping and it has absolutely helped. I'm so glad that moving is helping as opposed to hindering. Staying fit has been so controversial to my friends and family but I know it's essential for me.

Poppyseed has also started kicking pretty high up in my belly, just under my ribs. So far these are not uncomfortable, but I hear through the grapevine that such kicks can become quite painful. She's worth it.

Other than that the compliments continue to pour in. I wonder do all pregnant women receive these? People seem fascinated by pregnancy and even though I may feel utterly rough, others seem to see a glow. Pregnancy certainly brings out the generous side of people. No wonder some women go on to have a dozen kids, they are addicted to the attention. It is really very lovely however and very timely as right now I feel less than glowing. Such compliments will buoy me through the ungraceful waddling third trimester. Fourteen weeks to go. Poppyseed is the size of a cucumber; cool as they say.

16 February 2012

I'm feeling slightly down on myself today. Yesterday I had an irrational reaction to something James said. Whilst it's easy to blame pregnancy hormones, I don't think that's the case. I know myself well enough to blame good, old-fashioned insecurity. Yep, I got a few insecurities yet to be booted out by my spiritual styling. Not as many as most, but I've definitely got them. And they aren't pretty. Insecurities pop out of a pleasant day and turn everything grey; the worst thing about them is the way they manifest.

Instead of recognizing the insecurity as my problem it's natural to see the person who triggered the insecurity as the one to blame, but James is not to blame. He said something entirely devoid of intention and I acted like he was attempting to destroy me and then lauded on about how insensitive he was being. This was really only to deflect from the fact of what my brain was doing. A tiny part of me knew I was being ridiculous, but the insecure part, trampled over the top of her and pointed to the culprit as being James. We had a few cross words and this blew the steam out of my kettle. I quickly realized I had nowhere to go with my argument, backed down and apologized. I've felt silly ever since.

Dear Poppyseed,
I've been doing some thinking, my love. Thinking about people, about how we can so easily decide to dislike a whole gender, race, religion or cultural background simply because of one experience, because of one bad thing. I was brought up to see all people as equals. I want you to see that too.

I will be honest with you. Some of us, as a species, behave in a manner that is vile, hostile or cruel. Such folk are doubtless this way because of vileness perpetrated to them and suffering they have borne in life. Vileness is most often accumulated through experience; we are not born that way. Most people mean well. They really do. From the bottom of their hearts they are doing the best they can in what is a very tricky life. But we all have our experiences; we all have little segments of our lives that mess us up. Some more than others, some folks are sadly beyond repair.

We are all human beings stepping through this world with our own baggage and burdens. Some are kind, some are cruel, some are a little bit of both depending on what time of day you catch them. All you can do is be as good and kind as you can, forgive others and use your intuition to steer you clear of trouble and troublesome folk.

Life can be a hard slog and holding onto limited, prejudiced beliefs makes it even harder. So trust your instinct my baby, be brave and love everyone for who they are, because we all, deep down, deserve it. Love people for their errors and mistakes because from them they and we can choose to grow. We need not allow people to hurt us again and again, but we can take meaning from when they did, and be grateful that the pain we suffered has made us who we are, and made us less likely to suffer it again. Life is a funny little lesson and all that we meet - good and bad – are our teachers. So let them teach and know that you teach them back. Take what matters from each study session and abandon the rest. Be brave, my girl and use your heart, and for as long as I can I will try to be your most sensible guide.

Love, Mum

17 February 2012

This morning I took James to work, but before leaving the house, I noticed that Jimi cat was acting suspiciously by the front door. I got down on my hands and knees to locate his latest victim, during which time Jimi, thinking I'd joined the hunt, purred loudly and rolled over to let Alpha Cat Alice have a swipe at his prey. I spotted the tiniest little face squeezed tight into a few centimeters under the doorframe and my heart sank. It was 5am, and I knew that upon dropping James off I'd have to then commence operation Vole Rescue, before I could get some extra sleep.

I dropped a blanket over the door bottom to try and hide poor Mr Vole from Jimi and set off to take James. All the way to and from dropping James at work, I pleaded with the universal powers that be to make the rescue efforts easy. I really didn't want to spend the morning in pursuit of a tiny four-legged whirlwind.

On returning home I found that Jimi had moved the blanket, but Mr Vole was nowhere to be seen. Jimi looked perplexed. I decided to bundle up the blanket and shake it outside, just in case Voley was hidden in it. As I did this not one, but two baby voles dropped out and scuttled off! Who knew that Jimi was starting a collection! But for my part all I can say is, universe thank you for sparing the voles – and thank you for letting me get my sleep. You work in funny ways, but when you work, you rock.

18 February 2012
I've been at my Mum's house since yesterday, just having a lovely time, relaxing and resting. I found it a little hard to slow down and was threatening to wash my car earlier, but after a pedicure and massage at Mum's local salon I decided instead to treat myself to a long, hot bath. So long in fact that Mum became concerned for my welfare and needed to shout up and check I still existed!

It's been really nice to be away from the never-ending dust at home and to do nothing except watch films and feel my baby kick. I spoke with my American grandparents today too; it was lovely to chat about their first great grandchild! I'm their first grandchild and Mum was their first child. Three generations of first females!

James has a singer in the studio today. He called me up whilst she was recording and we had a lovely chat. When you live with someone it can be refreshing to be away from them and communicate differently. I loved that phone call, it felt nice to be remembered and thought of. When you are together all the time being thought of is unavoidable, but getting a call when you are apart, can reignite that spark of 'I miss you' even after ten years together.

Right now, James and I are exploring new ground, a whole new version of 'loved up'. It's not loved up in a romantic or sexy sense. It's more a 'big ass commitment' and 'serious baby creation' and 'trust and honor' sense. We are co-creators in a miracle and that is beautiful, serious, crazy and wonderful. I guess we are partners in life, literally.

After ten years, I adore that fella. Thank god for him, and everything we've been through together, so much stuff, great, good and horrendous too. I've spent more of my life with him than I have many other people. In the past year, I feel a far deeper connection has come about. Prior to that we loved each other, had fun, got silly, got crazy, but, whether we really fully connected I'm not sure... Of course we did connect in moments, or else ten years would have been tedious. But this year, for reasons, some unknown, some known, we have really and truly found each other. That is perhaps because we have finally found ourselves. And I know that Miss Poppyseed has helped on that path too.

I would usually think that no other person could make you change or make you more self-aware. However in this instance, I think perhaps they can. The awaited arrival of a little baby can most definitely help you to see yourself clearly, if, of course, you want to. This has been the first of Miss P's many challenges to her parents. '*Quick, find yourselves; I'm on my way*', she has whispered from my womb.

I am looking forward to seeing my James tomorrow. As my third trimester swiftly approaches, I'm suddenly keen to cocoon him and I into a land of cuddles, snuggles and conversations with belly. I need to nest. As he has nearly finished decorating the house, we are on track for baby bonding, hand holding, back stroking, serious adult only couch sitting, lovely time. Whilst we still can. I want to get our bond as strong as possible so that Poppyseed comes home to a fully bonded pair of parents. I want to fill the house with the vibe of love, trust and friendship. So yeah, I can't wait to see my man tomorrow.

20 February 2012

I must have had an adverse reaction to staying in a different bed at my Mum's house. I spent the afternoon in hip/back agony. I came home and after doing some very light housework, I was compelled to lie down on the bed and recover. James has exhausted himself from the weekend of decorating and late nights doing music in his loft studio, Mabbey Road. The result being that he snored badly all last night, did half a day at work today, came home, and snored all afternoon. So much for our romantic reunion! We are like a couple of gnarled old people who need to rest.

This morning I wrote my first non-spiritual blog for the *Huffington Post*. Indeed, this time I wrote about fashion, well maternity fashion. Leggings to be precise, and the fact that they are the only clothing I am comfortable in, but the last thing I want to be wearing. It was fun to write something different, so a rant based around my embracing of leggings was perfect...

"I woke this morning with a feverish compulsion to write about leggings, maternity leggings to be specific. Though the slant was veering towards the poor choices available in budget shopping for pregnant ladies. Please excuse me, I am no fashion writer, I'm a spiritual writer who 'suffers' shopping and all things consumer driven, so for me to turn my words to this, something must be terribly wrong in the world. Either that, or the pregnancy hormones have finally gotten to me. Humor me, let me attend to this rant and I am convinced that the pregnant amongst us may rally to my cries.

Prior to my now seven months of pregnancy I had a moment of passion where I decided I must throw away all of my leggings, even the wet look ones which upon first wearing had seemed so very radical. I packed them off to the charity shop knowing that dozens of girls, younger than myself, would be astounded by this true find in amongst the old lady sweaters. I proudly declared myself a legging-free zone.

Leggings, it seems to me, are the last bastions of the lazy dresser. They cover our legs in regulation style, can be dressed down and up and serve the very basic necessity of 'clothing' quite adequately. Yet in spite of this adequacy I simply had to break free. My heart lay elsewhere, I'm no fashion expert, but I figured that dresses, fitted trousers, lovely jeans were preferable to skin tight black coverings whereby if you stare to close you may just see some flesh, or, god forbid, a hair missed in waxing.

Yet something terrible has happened. Not only have I reverted to type, I now own two pairs of the devilishly comfortable monstrosity that are maternity leggings. And the reason why? Well maternity clothing on a budget is truly dire. I expected to be bowled over by choice, for it is 2012, and the newspapers are choc full of pregnant debutantes looking classy, sassy and fine. Though, if I'm honest, I see more leggings on these ladies than I do on the pins of other non-pregnant famous faces. I may be wrong, but didn't Beyonce grace a pair or two whilst carrying her baby? If Miss B had to endure the ravages of soft and cozy lycra, then what hope is there for the rest of the world?

I have three months of pregnancy left, and I am not prepared to spend on items that rot so quickly or that will look ridiculous come the end of May. The shopping time and hours spent in changing rooms is likely to damage my already hormonal mental health, perhaps beyond repair. Having perused the websites of so many high street fashion stores, I can only find maternity clothes determined to make me look bland, dull and inexcusably mumsy. So why even bother taking my rattling pregnant pelvis to the streets?

It's become so desperate, that recently I almost online-purchased a pair of maternity leopard print leggings. I know, I know, it's against everything I'm fighting for, but they were the only thing that had any semblance of personality about them, any semblance of being just a little bit rock 'n' roll. Then I imagined the inevitable thinned out look of stretched and over-worn leopard print and decided to take the soulful approach. I slipped back into my pajamas and didn't leave the house. Perhaps this is the only answer?

I am so outside of my league in this debate, that I'm not even sure if there is a debate? I do know however that Vivienne Westwood has struck out at modern throwaway fashion, saying we all look the same and that seventy-year-old ladies could teach us a trick or two. Well my Grandma is ninety and her staple outfit for the last twenty years has been navy, a navy blouse and navy trousers, the occasional blush of pink lips on a fancy occasion. She looks good, she has found her niche. My Gran knows horses more than she does fashion but I'm sure she would tell you that leggings are simply jodhpurs for walking. Jodhpurs that would not hold up to more than a few meters at the Grand National before they split, laddered and became suitable only for your Halloween wenches costume.

As for me, I think I have given up. Other than my brother's wedding in March when I may well have to make some sincere efforts, I am going to become wholly reliant on what I already own, sandwiched with occasional legging abuse. The classic 'dress with leggings' look is something I intend to own. I feel I have no choice. I will continue to lament the preposterous lack of choice in fair priced maternity clothing as I lounge in my horridly comfortable black over the bumps. Indeed I will of course do all I can to remind myself of everything spiritual, that fashion is a load of bunkum and the most important thing is the baby growing in my belly. Which is all madly, deeply true. I will consent to embracing the leggings for now and I shall allow them to serve a purpose. In three months time, they will be honorably discharged, screwed up, tied in knots and gifted to George my rabbit who has a psychopathic streak for scraps of material and will be sure to treat them with the vicious disdain they deserve."

Dear Poppyseed,
I should now be addressing you as 'Dear Cauliflower' as that is apparently how big you are. But it doesn't have the same ring to it! I hope you are doing well and are snuggled up warm inside me. I know I've been on a little bit of an emotional roller coaster lately, I sure hope it hasn't bothered you too much. Whilst it may be good practice for life, you really don't need to go there yet!

My belly bump is getting so much bigger. I stroke you all the time. I can't help it, I'm twenty-seven weeks pregnant today, which means thirteen weeks until I see your face.

In two weeks, Dad and I are taking our baby-moon. A weekend in the country, just us. Oh, and the cats too. They are coming so that Nana Bev can help us with decorating. The decorating here has been manic. Your Dad is exhausted and I'm tired from just observing... So your lovely Nana is taking over and letting Poppa and I escape for a few days. Bless her heart; she's a good woman. She's going to love you so very much, she already does. Your name is stamped on her heart. It's Nana Bev's mother you will be named after. So maybe there will be a special bond there. I hope so.

Love, Mum

23 February 2012
Last night it was so lovely to see my best friends! Reina is looking fabulously pregnant now with a full on bump. She has eight weeks left and it's all so ridiculously exciting. She looks adorable. It was refreshing to be so focused on somebody else's bump.

I came home to a very stressed out young James. You can't leave these blokes alone for one minute! Work had gotten to him; on top of everything else he has been throwing himself in to, such as decorating, and being strong for me. He felt like he couldn't cope and so I sat him down to explain that he both can and he does, but that blips in mood are occasional and inevitable. Take my up and down pregnancy as a prime example of such blips!

But on a dark February night wise words can go out of the window in the face of life's pressures. So we had a big heart to heart. In the past, we may have rowed. I may have been impatient or critical, but somewhere in the past year I've changed too. All I could see was a soul I love having a hard day. When you see a person's weakness, and their strength, and you truly believe in them, there is no space for fighting, nagging or bickering, and whilst we will always bicker (of course), this was not the time for it.

Compassion gets you much further in life. Everything is better now. An hour's blip is water under the bridge and sometimes quite helpful as it shows how far a person has come. Falling back into a chasm, even temporarily, shows you precisely where you don't want to be. All things are constructive. Life is an education, life without blips would be a life misunderstood.

I just want to rave a little while about my other soul mate, Molly, my cat. Since working from home we are inseparable. She is my shadow and I am hers. I love that little cat with so much heart and soul. She's my angel, she has taken to sleeping on me all night. She accompanies my billions of nighttime toilet trips. I feel she is watching out for me, being my friend. Before baby arrives I know I'll have to stop the sleeping on me situation, it's not safe, but for now it's a lovely little habit that I welcome. She makes me feel so safe and loved. I've had so many cats before, cats I have loved madly, but Molly is The One. I can't think how I'll ever see past her. She is my soul-cat, my puddy-wuddy best friend. I wonder if she knows I'm pregnant? If she does I hope she is happy for it. I often joke that Poppyseed's first word will be Molly, her name is mentioned so much around here. I'm so looking forward to introducing my two girls and I hope they too can be in love with each other.

24 February 2012
Had a midwife's appointment with Jo and she asked how I was feeling. I said I'd been fine but on occasion 'a bit moody', the response was a very surprised 'only a bit?'

She has a point. It feels like I have a few wonderful days with great moods, and energy, then I drop straight out of that into something far more despondent. Today I was okay until I had to go to the supermarket. It felt like everyone was gunning for me and that my bump was target number one for trolleys and people to bang into. I noticed how massively unaware most of the supermarket shoppers were of anyone in their vicinity. I felt as though I was running a dangerous gauntlet. That, and there were no suitable lunches for a knocked up girl like me. This pretty much tipped me over into foul mood territory. From there I then managed to block the pin on my debit card and I think that at this point steam released itself from my ears. Back home now and I feel fine again.

Could this be the start of some pregnancy agoraphobia? If so, I hope it comes and goes with pregnancy. James and I are out tonight to see a friend's band play. I am dreading it. Busy, drunken crowds of people who are even less self-aware than the blinkered supermarket shoppers. I feel that I have to go though. We will only be out an hour or so and I know James would like it, so I'm doing it for him. Truthfully though, I can't think of anything worse right now, but love is as love does and James deserves an hour's break from our sofa and film routine.

...I wound myself up all day about tonight. I went to pick James up and burst into tears about being seven months pregnant and all the reasons I felt uncomfortable going out tonight. He was such a sweetie, he wasn't one bit bothered and repeatedly told me that I didn't need to keep explaining myself. He wasn't interested in my reasons for not wanting to go out. He simply accepted that

I didn't want to. Love is as love does. Clearly that works both ways. Love that man.

26 February 2012

We went baby window-shopping today. I stood totally lost in the middle of a melee of prams and got the giggles. I didn't have a clue what I was looking at. It all seemed suddenly very grown up and unexpected. James went and accosted an assistant and it was soon all explained, so a new education in baby accessories begins…

It was a cute trip. Sweetly, James got ever so emotional when he saw a baby grow that said, 'Daddy and Mummy plus me equals Three'. This in turn made me emotional, and a random trip to look at products turned extra special.

I did an hour yoga session in the gym on Friday, but when it comes to bending over and putting on clothes I become exhausted. I was planning on making gardening my new hobby during maternity leave, but half an hour's gardening yesterday was a killer. I guess for now little trips to the garden are sufficient.

I do love gardening. When I've been in the garden I feel grounded, relaxed and happy. After a gardening session, I close my eyes and all I see is shoots, leaves and branches. It's as if I become at one with Momma Earth and she gets inside me. I come from a line of gardening lovers. My Mum and my Grandma adore it to the point of addiction and I can see me getting that way inclined too. My Grandma's letters from America used to amuse me as a child as they were really just gardening reports, the last thing a kiddy wants to read! My brothers and I used to giggle as Mum read to us the full-on essays about what was growing, and what birds had visited. I guess she has the gardening bug big time. It doesn't seem so funny now I'm grown up; it seems beautiful, earthy, and shamanic.

Maybe in her time, Poppyseed will develop a love for all things that grow, I'll be certain to give her a little patch of her very own to experiment with. I will do my best to make the garden a beautiful, safe place for her. One of my main memory themes from childhood is gardens. Our garden at my first home, Granny in the USA's garden, Granny in the UK's garden. Gardens are magical places. I used to try to sneak up on birds and I'd always be taking grass and water to Mr Lion – the stone lion who lived in the rockery. Gardens are fertile playgrounds of imagination and whilst the garden we have in my current home is small, it is still perfect for memories to be hatched.

27 February 2012
I had a wonderful freaky dream last night that we could see Poppyseed through my belly. I could grab her feet and hands and see her big green eyes looking out at us.

This morning has been odd. There has been some stuff going on with people I know and I've been sat listening to a heap of terribly judgmental bitching and gossip. When I tried to counter the bitching, I was shot down. I tried to defend the person being spoken of and instead provoked further assaults on that person's character. This was meant, I guess, to defend the bitches and to justify their bitching, but it's just ugly, mean and petty. I have of course dosed out my fair share of bitchiness in my time, I'm not innocent in this respect. But a few years ago I put a pin in it. Whilst I love a bit of gossip, I steer clear of the vindictive, catty form of it.

People revel in bitching, they report back tragic, messy stuff about others lives in such a self-righteous way, and too often with a smirk on their face. I don't care what a person has done; character assassination is no longer my style. People do things good and bad, but most often, they only do them because in that instance they hope it will make them happy. I get that talking about other people's lives and choices is fascinating. Of course it is. But being judgmental about their lives and choices is where I believe we should draw the line. Our choices are for us to deal with and learn from, not for others to use as bullets against us. My opinion remains that life is hard, life is hard, and life is hard. Nasty bitching and gossip has no place in making it easier.

I was proud of myself today. Proud that I felt uncomfortable about what was said. I'm proud that Poppyseed won't hear that type of talk from me. I'm proud that she'll be brought up with an understanding of sympathy, empathy and forgiveness.

Dear Poppyseed
Don't let anyone tell you that women are the worst for bitching. Don't believe it for a second. Both genders love a good old spiteful gossip. Indeed, I've seen some of the worst bitching of my life come from grown men who should know better. Put it this way, the Leicester music scene (full of dudes) could give *The Real Housewives* a run for their money!

I truly hope that no one will ever speak badly of you, but it's likely that they will. Humans love to chat about one another, and often they love to be less than flattering. They take something small you did and exaggerate, and worse than that they judge you. As if they themselves were so damn perfect. If this happens to you, my little love, you must hold your head proud. Do not allow the callous comments to enter your heart. You are not what other people say you are, nor are you defined by your choices or mistakes. Your choices are an offshoot of the deeper you and your mistakes are no worse than anyone else's. It is your mistakes that will hone and craft you into the best little lady you can be, so embrace them.

I do understand that mean comments and name-calling are hard to deal with; they cut harder and faster than anything else. They go on beyond the schoolyard too. Callous words can break your heart and stick with you a lifetime. But they mean very little. Someone's fleeting opinion of you is worth absolutely nothing, I promise you that. What do these people know of you? They cannot see your heart and soul.

At heart people who bitch are trying to deflect from their own choices and their own mistakes. As if painting their talk with stories and opinions about you will stop people realizing what they fear most about themselves. The bitchiest people are always the most insecure; the ones who want to create a smokescreen of superiority. Don't believe their superiority for a second. Truly powerful proud people do not involve themselves in the minutiae of silliness that is the office or school ground bitch-fest. See through their blabber and understand, compassionately, that the bitch is lacking something; there is a hole in them that idol chatter fills.

Bitching is a tactic to fill time and boost egos. It means nothing, not a thing. It is a stronghold of the weak and the powerless. To see beyond the bitchiness is to glimpse the good, sincere heart of all humanity, to ignore or hush the bitching is to empower ourselves with love and forgiveness and non-judgmental living. I can't protect you from either bitching yourself or being bitched about, all I can advise is steer clear, stay humble and know that people will always make mistakes – yourself included. You have no right to judge and no one has a right to judge you. It's happier simply to smile and accept, be true to the vast vat of love you have in your soul for all people and all things.

Know that from mistakes we can all grow and so, nobody is deserving of horrific words said in their name. We do the best that we can in the moment. Know this and free yourself from the chains of persecution that bitchiness is. Bite your tongue and choose to see the best. Be a real friend, not a backstabber. Be confident in who you are becoming and offer love by embracing everyone's mistakes, problems, errors or otherwise. None of us are perfect. Live and Let Live. Know always too that no matter what may be said about you, you are always utterly, heart-stoppingly perfect to me.

Love always, Momma

29 February 2012

Today, thus far, has been a big weird memory fest. I've been inundated by thoughts of my past. Plus there is more decorating happening this weekend as me and James go away and leave Nana Bev to it.

I decided to get all the papers from around my desk and recycle as much as possible. It was a confounding experience. I felt hugely disconnected to parts of my life and easily tore up letters, notes and diaries for recycling, some of them, symbolically I placed in the bin. Memories of all kinds flooded over me, it's funny what we keep… In the end much more than I expected was discarded. In part I wanted to do away with excess, but also with things that no longer represent me and things that quite frankly I don't want Poppyseed to ever see.

Being a writer, I have written a lot down over the years. Whilst most people have fleeting thoughts, now forgotten, I found some real pearls of negativity stored up within the folds of my paperwork. True as they may be at the time I wrote them, they have no place in this home now. So they went. Indeed, so did a lot of my spiritual diaries. When I was in the deep throes of being overtly 'spiritual' I consulted cards often, had readings done and wrote what I perceived to be messages from Spirit. Looking back through that I felt no attachment. Any messages I did receive were for then, and not for now, so that all went too. I am so less reliant on a spiritual existence for advice these days and rarely ever touch an angel card, never mind a tarot card. Not because I don't believe, because I do, but because at this time of my life I am thrilled to be in the moment. As such readings, prophecies and spiritual accoutrements are not something I feel drawn to.

Of course I kept a lot too. Cuttings of my writings, old poems, letters to long dead cats. I'm not without sentiment for my past. I probably managed to cut the junk in half and James will have a challenge taking the bins out tonight.

Three months to go. The third trimester begins today, eighty-four sleeps, twelve weeks, it's crazy stuff. I started to really think forward to the hypnobirthing classes, labor even. Since my belly has emerged and Poppyseed is now kicking all the time I feel much more ready to be a Mommy. Pregnancy is definitely a process I have needed. It's been like therapy and I'm sure it will continue to be so for the next eighty-four days. Following that I guess we turn a whole new corner. Adventure awaits.

✡

3 March 2012

James and I embarked on our baby moon this weekend. We booked three nights away in a cottage on a farm in the Peak District. It was all very quaint and pretty. Unfortunately the cottage housed the worlds most uncomfortable sofas, so our plan to vegetate was hampered somewhat. But otherwise the break was much needed.

On our first full day in the cottage the farmer told me that a baby cow had been born that morning. We went to visit the new family and were honored (and a little grossed out) to watch Momma cow eat the placenta. Whilst I don't intend to eat my placenta, this made me feel so connected to Daisy. She too was a Momma, this was her fourteenth calf, and so she was an experienced Momma. It was a beautiful sight. I found the whole scene very moving, Momma cow, brand new calf sharing a barn with other Mommas and their babies.

Cows are no fools. They had a stunning wisdom and peacefulness about them. I had a little chat with them, as I do all animals, explaining that I meant no harm. I told them that I was going to be a momma too, that I just wanted to spend some time with them. They gazed back with their beautiful big brown eyes, so happy just to be there in the moment with their little ones. I'm so glad I'm a vegetarian, because if I weren't this moment would have ruined me. To witness the sentient, real love and understanding between these gorgeous creatures renders the ability to chow down on a burger null and void.

Later that night James and I were playing with his telescope examining the skies. When suddenly a comet/shooting star rode through the sky. Burning brightly all the way from far on our left to far on our right until it eventually burnt out. It was mad impressive and gave true meaning to all those overused terms mega, immense, epic, awesome. It had two trails coming off it at one point, like a giant fire in the sky. It was in our eye line for about fifteen seconds as a bright burning glow then as a smoky grey shadow evaporating into the night. Stunning.

I've researched such phenomena and watched a host of videos on line. What we witnessed was more than a regular shooting star. It was a meteor fireball. We were so lucky to have been out at that time, on that date and to see this rare occurrence. It felt like a blessing from above. That is how our ancestors would have seen it, as a sign, a blessing, and a good omen. So I choose to see it that way, a spectacular display of love from the heavens to our little baby and us.

I knew that day would be lucky because two white feathers were on the doorstep of the cottage in the morning. James had told me that he was outside when some birds flew overhead and the white feathers literally fell out of them to his feet. Another fabulous omen.

After a nice country weekend, we are back to reality and that reality is painted white. Whilst we were away James' mum Beverley kindly offered to paint our whole downstairs. She did so with a bad back and very little help, it looks fantastic. It is definitely a clean slate to build upon. Before it was cream and cluttered, which is fine, but clutter is magically attracted to baby's mouths. So all of that has to go. No more can I leave sweetie-sized crystals in corners to usher in good times via Feng Shui. No more can musical equipment clutter up the dining space. This is a whole new way of existence and it's exciting. From here on in 'stuff' is going in drawers, crystals must be out of reach and musical equipment can go in Mabbey Road upstairs.

7 March 2012

Belly is getting bigger. My belly button is almost flat now. James thinks it will pop out, I think not, perhaps we should take bets? We purchased our pram system today. Yes that's right, it's a whole system. Not quite so large as an eco system…but almost. I used to wrongly believe that a pram was a pram. Oh no. Prams have evolved. They are like the Transformers, but a pram is a car seat, a buggy, a stroller in disguise. We got an ex-display model from an auction site, which seemed a bargain, albeit an expensive one.

I'm feeling good in myself. Far less achy and creaky than I was, so I'm embracing it while it lasts. Tonight James and I will go to our first hypnobirthing session. It's a full on three hours. Whilst I've spent a lot of time in classes and spiritual groupings this will be new to James. He hasn't been in a class since school, which he left aged 16. I'm not sure how many classes he actually made it to back then either, spending most of his time in the music rooms! Despite being out of practice he seems to be looking forward to it. Not only will hypnobirthing help with labor it's chock full of life and relationship learning for parents to be. So...it's like group therapy then! Should be interesting.

Feeling less inclined to work at the moment and more inclined to potter, well potter and eat! Tempted, happily towards healthier foods, though chocolate and ice cream do still have an enigmatic pull.

Other than an achy back and on/off tiredness, I've never felt better. Perhaps it's abstention from alcohol, perhaps it's pregnancy itself, but I have never gone a whole winter without catching a cold, usually I get several colds, and yet here I am, it's March and I'm snot free. I've not taken so much as a paracetamol since August or September. I feel great, I know I have my down days, moodiness and exhaustion but I have truly been healthy. Pregnancy suits me. It's been fabulous. Of course it's not over yet. Eleven weeks to go and who knows what may lie ahead, but as I'm feeling good I say bring it on!

8 March 2012
Why does this happen?

Yesterday I felt great, happy go lucky and energetic. And as is becoming standard with me I rave about it in my diary. Then the next day I'm tired, grouchy and super emotional. What that's all about? On days like this anything can set off a flood of tears. Earlier today I felt overwhelmed, that brought on a teary session. Just now, James sent me a text saying, 'Love you Mummy' and the floodgates opened again.

To try to counter this rash of heady hot tears, I have purchased, and am listening to, classical relaxing music. I also painted my nails bright pink. It's not really helped. My concentration is out the window and work matters are dragging me down. It seems that everyone and their dog has some kind of issue with me right now, and as the day job involves managing complaints, I'm up against some really seasoned complainers. Normally it's water off a duck's back, but today it's frustrating. Working from home is not always ideal, and the distraction of office friends is much missed. James has already given me one pep talk and I hope I can snap out of it before he gets home. I have nothing to be down about, not really. I need to 'woman' up!

Last night was the first hypnobirthing class. I feel inspired by the session and empowered to overcome any childbirth fear to bring Poppyseed into the world peacefully. Hypnobirthing has transformed how I see birth. It is no longer a nerve inducing, painful torture that lies ahead, but an amazing powerful, feminine experience that will lead to the most precious gift I'll ever have. Looking at birth in this way suits my spiritual sentiments and is far preferable than living in fear of blood, guts and agony.

Hypnobirthing theory has absolutely given me a new approach and has eased this last bit of pregnancy. If I hadn't looked into it, I'm not sure where I would be now. I guess I'd be in a place of fear. Living from a place of fear would not be ideal for Baby Poppyseed or me. Being free from fear is beautiful. Looking forward to birth is not something I ever thought would happen. Feeling empowered is a whole other level I hadn't dreamt of in my wildest dreams. And yet I am, I'm looking forward with joy, excitement and with the knowing that birth can be my beautiful experience, I can own it, frame it and dress it up as I wish.

I wish to have a spiritual, peaceful, natural birth managed by breath, hypnotherapy, meditation, massage, water, music and aromatherapy. I don't want pain relief and I don't want to be in a hospital. I hope to go to a local birthing centre and keep everything as relaxed, natural and beautiful as I can. It's so exciting, to give the gift of a loving, peaceful birth to my little girl.

So yes, I'm feeling inspired. Though I believe that the three-hour session of full on concentration in class may have played some small part in today's grumps! Three hours of evening learning is a bit too much for pregnant old me right now.

9 March 2012
Yesterday I bought a classical music album especially for pregnancy. Today I'm sure little Poppyseed is dancing along. When we listen to it I can feel her inside me making beautiful baby butterfly shapes. What a precious feeling.

13 March 2012
An article I wrote about gay marriage and parenting went a little bit global. I won't lie, it was lovely to have the attention to my writing even if some of it was negative. I realized that I'm stronger than I was a few years back. I remember my first ever experience of public criticism with a cringe. Somebody referred to me as a 'Spiritual Barbie' and it really upset me. This new article has attracted a host of malevolent and personal attacks on me. I found them funny. This shows some good progression on my backbone. Here it is anyway…

"I was born and initially raised by a handsome stable of hetero-sexuality. Dad was the local church vicar, Mum his loyal wife. My playground was the extensive vicarage with views of a graveyard. I was a good girl who refused to snack on the body of Christ, even when offered. I knew I wasn't old enough. Life was all sunshine and loveliness.

Then real life struck. Like many children before and after me, my parents divorced. Daddy was to become a 'writer' needing his own space, whilst Mummy moved in with a woman. Life never looked different. My main devastation in all this was that I had to leave my beloved Brownie troop. It didn't occur to me that the lesbian partnership I was about to be raised by was anything less than normal.

The weirdest thing about my childhood was probably when Dad turned his back on the church and became a Pagan High Priest. I was taken aside and point blank informed, "Alice, I'm a Pagan."

My blood pumped faster as I anticipated being the focal point of a virgin sacrifice. This was not to pass. Paganism was all very intriguing for a young teenage girl - think tarot cards, meditation and vegetarian feasts. I met a lot of pre-emo Goths and Punks, I was allowed to drink red wine and I developed a penchant for men with long hair. It added to my teenage years in glorious fashion. Upon learning healing skills I fixed a dying gerbil. Buffy and Bella eat your heart out!

Compared to this the lesbian duoship that was my weekday parentage was rather boring. The relationship lasted 10 years, which was sufficient to see me through to adulthood, breaking up eventually due to good old-fashioned human flaws. I know that the parentage tried their best, I was loved and they provided all I needed materially. We had pets, we did kooky family stuff such as putting on plays and pretending to be Mr Bean. I had chicken soup when poorly. We went on long country rambles, ate roast dinners on a Sunday and until I was considered old enough I was not allowed to watch anything above my age certificate, or, for that matter *EastEnders*.

The only downfall to this gay parenting model was the discrimination and prejudice visited on us by members of the local community. As kids we would often fall out with the neighbors children. Whenever this happened their parents would threaten to call social services over our unusual parenting arrangement. This was heartbreaking and scary. I once confided in a friend about my lesbian mum and she promised not to tell, but then on occasion, tried to use her silence to bribe me. Funnily enough Facebook tells me she is gay herself now!

I learned not to talk about it. My brothers did talk about it, and their experience was less than pleasant. However this was a sign of the times, of ignorance, prejudice and the cruelty of other people. Had my gay parents been allowed to be married and made 'normal', some of the crueler facets of my youth may not have occurred. My experience is that society caused me more problems than the parenting itself. Because isn't it true that all parents mess you up, or make you happy, and that this is irrespective of gender, sexuality, race, religion or any other tick box. Isn't that just the nature of parenting?

Being recognized by society as 'equal' is of far more benefit to gay households, than the steamy fluff pouring out of the mouths of people such as Cardinal O'Brien. His war cries against 'grotesque' gay marriage are the same thing I heard all my youth, the fishwife next door, the teasing kids, the fear of the different. They are meaningless, they do not come from God, they come from dogma, religious blinkers and ignorance.

My experience tells me that marriage and relationships are very simple. They are about two people, messed up in their own unique ways, trying to make a place for themselves in the world.

Heterosexual union certainly cannot be claimed to fly any flag on perfection. From my practical and spiritual perspective I believe that our individual flaws are often made most apparent through our relationships formalized or otherwise. It is from here that we can work at improving ourselves, at making our life, and the lives of other people happier. From entering into partnership with another the most we can hope for is some happiness, some learning, some place to call home. Gay, straight or otherwise, there is nothing 'grotesque' about that."

The most common comment to me this week is how big I've got. A tiny paranoid voice in my head tells me that this means more than just my bump, perhaps people are simply calling me fat. My mummy parts, boobs and tummy, are huge. I'm sure the rest is pretty much normal. Still…as a woman (no matter how spiritual) it's not easy being told all the time how big and massive and huge I am. I'll be careful not to say that to other mums to be. Or If I do, I'll be specific about which part of them I'm referring too.

15 March 2012

It's my brother Mike's wedding this weekend. He lives in Tokyo, where he met his beautiful Korean girlfriend, Su Young. As a result, they are having what I call the Worldwide Wedding Tour. A wedding in Tokyo for friends, one in Korea for Su Young's family and then the grand finale in Birmingham, England for us lot. I'm so excited to see them and for one of us to actually get wed proper. James and I ran off to Vegas for ours, which was great fun, but this is full-on church, white dress and disco after; the whole shebang! Thrice!

Today I went for the day to Mum's house to meet up with Mike and Su Young and my youngest brother Joe and his lady, Vicky. I organized for us girls to go to a spa this afternoon as a small hen party. It was really lovely and relaxing. As Su Young and Vicky have never met before it was good for that to happen so that Su Young could feel that she had some girly friends at her wedding.

It's totally manic at my Mum's with Mike and Su Young's worldwide wedding preparations. I'm feeling pretty good in myself. I woke up with a cold but had a word with the cosmic forces and stated that I was not prepared to accept that right now. I went back to sleep for two hours and it's vanished. Great magicky stuff. At night, I headed home after a hilarious family dinner together. I needed my own bed. However being with my whole family whilst our newest member brews in my tummy made it all the more special. As my brother lives in Japan this is the first time he will meet my baby bump, and he won't see her again until she is born and quite a few months old. So this time together is precious.

16 March 2012
I have been reading the book, *Ina May's Guide to Childbirth*, by the birthing force to be reckoned with, Ina May Gaskin. Ina May runs a natural birthing centre in Tennessee and is renowned for assisting Women to have incredible, natural births. She has a low rate of any kind of intervention and she returns the power of birth to Mothers and Women tenfold. This book is an inspiration. It pulls no punches either. Some of the births sound fraught, difficult, painful and intense. But what they all have in common is that each one becomes so empowering, so incredible, and so damned beautiful. This book is a love story to the idea of bringing a little one into the world naturally. I so hope that I can achieve this. If only I could afford flights to Tennessee...so tempting!

19 March 2012
I've had the loveliest weekend. Mike and Su Young's wedding was the best wedding I have ever been to. I felt happy inside and out, literally surrounded by encircling family. I felt so blessed to be a part of such warmth and so proud to be bringing Poppyseed into a world where these lovely people exist.

Family is so important. I've not always been the most family focused person, but I know that is changing. After this weekend I want to be sure Miss P grows up knowing everyone and having family in close reach.

In my childhood I was far removed from distant family as they lived overseas or long train journeys away. Family was never on tap, but I do hope this will be different for my little one. Even with people living in far-flung countries, it's important to keep closeness, even if some years that is only by Skype or email.

I've spent a few years discovering myself, writing books for an audience of strangers, but now I hope to draw my attention inward and to my nearest and dearest.

Mike and Su Young's wedding was a truly happy day. I didn't stop smiling and here lies some kind of key to my spiritual life; just being happy, being loved, being free of all the tags and labels that are unnecessary and maybe trying something different on for size. This past weekend, I was simply a family member and a mum-to-be and it's the happiest I've been in a very long while. I wasn't an author, a publisher or a tarot reader. I was just me, a person who fits into a family, without having to do anything, without wearing any kind of cap or detailed signature. Just me.

In spite of all this good times and familial insight the wedding has exhausted me. I was up at 8am for hair and in bed for 1am after helping to clean up a little. The middle bit involved assisting the bride, going on mad bow-tie seeking journeys to the neighbors, gave an emotional reading in church where I started blubbing within seconds and struggled to speak. I then declared myself pregnant and emotional to the audience. I managed to get through it, but Kahil Gibran, the author I was reading, has a lot to answer for. Following this, I danced, chatted, ate, toasted the happy couple with one tiny sip of champagne and generally made merriment.

We were joined at the wedding by Sue, our wedding's resident midwife. She kindly agreed to palpate my tummy. She showed me, James and the Grandmas-to-be which bit of baby was what. So we all had a gentle push and prod of little Poppyseed, which helped make her very much a part of the day.

As a result of all the excitement on Sunday, I was truly

wrecked. I've not felt this pregnantly tired since the first trimester. I slept in the afternoon and then watched TV all evening like a zombie. I have woken today a little better but vastly more aware of my growing bump. Poppyseed has certainly made herself known these past few days – revenge for all the palpating she endured at the wedding! I enjoy her wiggly, kicking company, but trips to the toilet have been frequent.

I have a radio interview to do shortly, but then I'm on wind down. I've closed down my social network Soul Café and my focus is much more internal. Soul Café was a great little social spot on the web that I started, but it often felt that I was putting out a lot with little return. I don't give to receive, but in this instance I was draining myself. I'll stay in contact with many of the people from Soul Café, but I know that when we close a door others will open. I am anticipating that. Life is very true to that phrase…so let's see what takes the space that Soul Café once held… But for now, full on hibernation and birth preparation starts after this last interview.

20 March 20012
Last night was fraught with weird pregnancy stress dreams. I can't remember the details but vaguely recall Liam Gallagher being there and him being a horrific bully. I believe I may have rescued a young maiden from his evil clutches, but can't quite recall the details. It was a good night's sleep in spite of dreams and the constant need to pee. It seems that sometimes having a pee makes me feel I need the toilet even worse. I'm learning to ignore the urination cravings as so often they are false. Hopefully this approach will not all end in tears and wet panties.

I had a moment today where I realized how much I'll miss being pregnant. It is such an all-consuming event in my life and I love carrying little baby with me everywhere. Last night, James and I were cuddling on the sofa when I had the realization that Poppyseed will be a baby soon, not just a bump. Seven and a half months into pregnancy and you would of thought I'd have figured that out already. But I've spent so much time bonding with her little soul, I forgot the obvious, she is more than a soul, she's a little physical being. This sentient soul is going to be sucking on my nipples and pooping in her nappy. What a realization!

Anyway I will miss pregnancy, I'll miss eating all kinds of things and adventuring in food for health. Whilst I can do that, pregnant or otherwise, it feels more worthy knowing it's for Poppyseed. I'll miss doing workouts and sending her to sleep. I'll miss her kicks and squiggles.

Pregnancy has been the most powerful and delicious experience of my life so far. It's just so...real. In a world of false, fraud and fancy packaging, there is something hugely beautiful and empowering about being a lady with child. I'm so pleased we embarked on this adventure. I will savor the next nine weeks and one day. I may never do this again and so whilst I'm still pregnant, it is my wonderful world.

21 March 2012

I took James driving last night. It was fun! I got him insured on the car for a month whilst he is learning to drive. He is having official lessons too. Which is a good job because having passed my test many years ago, he is constantly telling me things that I am getting wrong. Getting James driving is another ingredient of the 'baby pie'. Having lived in the same town all his life, and near to his work, he hasn't needed to drive. Then, when he got a job further afield, it was in the same far-flung little town that I worked in. So I'd drive him in. But my office no longer exists, so I can't take him to work anymore, and besides, I won't want to when we have the baby. Him getting a license can be prolonged no longer.

Poor James must be exhausted though. This 'baby pie' has called upon him to put forward a whole heap of ingredients. It's amazing what that man has achieved in the past few months. He has completely transformed his life and our house. I know he gets exhausted as a result and doing loads of overtime at work doesn't help him, but he's a real trooper and I want Poppyseed to know it, so here it is in black and white: Daddy is a Hero!

Last night I again had horrible dreams, I woke up with a mad craving for a chocolate croissant. I have nipped out to get one and it's just in the oven now. Last night was chocolate ice cream; it is clearly chocolate craving week. I can live with that! In the early days of pregnancy, chocolate made me feel so sick, even one small nibble would render me nauseous for an hour. Thankfully that didn't last.

I'm putting together a song list for Poppyseed with songs chosen for her by family and friends. I'm calling it 'Welcome to the World'. I was listening to my chosen song '*Carry You*' by Tori Amos and after the first chord, I was sobbing. I mean really blubbing my little heart out. I felt reluctant to let go of Miss P. I just want to keep her wrapped up safe in my belly. I even went so far as to worry about her when she is older and when James and I die. I know that's so morbid. But I've never been in a position before where someone really, really needs me. It's intense and the thought that I may not always be here for her is heartbreaking. Whatever happens I'm determined my spirit will stay with her. Forever and always. I'll find a way to be with her.

I never expected this level of emotion without having physically met my lady, I adore her. This is primal, spiritual, physical, mental and divine all wrapped up together and churning in my gut. She is challenging my heartstrings and they are playing for her and her alone.

22 March 2012

Last night was the second hypnobirthing class. I love it! It is such a great experience for us to undertake in getting ready for Poppyseed. I really don't understand how some folks make no preparation whatsoever and just turn up on the day freaked out and at the mercy of the establishment.

Hypnobirthing is such a hugely awesome holistic approach to birthing and babies. It's very exciting. A few things have arisen that need addressing though.

First I had asked my best friend Roisin to attend the birth with us. I guess I should ask my Mum, and/or James's mum, and I very nearly did, but decided that Roisin would be a better support for James, as they get on so well. So we risked upsetting both our mums, and had asked Rosh instead.

However this is all irrelevant now as we have decided it's better to just be James and me. Hypnobirthing has shown us how important it is to keep the birth intimate, much like the act that got us pregnant in the first place! Whilst I know Rosh would play a wonderful part and I love her dearly, we just don't feel right about it anymore. When I explained this to her she totally understood. She told me that she half expected that to happen anyway once James and I had gotten our heads around what was due to happen…

Secondly, James and I really want to focus on family bonding in the first two weeks after Poppyseed's birth. We need it to be just us three for most of the time. This may cause problems with all the lovely well wishers, but we feel strongly that this period is the only time we will get to know each other and settle in, especially as men only get two weeks paternity leave. We don't want this disturbed by answering the door, being polite or having anyone buzzing around us being helpful. I know how harsh this sounds, particularly against our own Mothers, but after two weeks they can be involved all the time. But for the two week baby-moon while James is on paternity leave, we need space. And of course we will see some people, such as the Mothers, we won't totally refuse access to baby. But we just need to manage and monitor what does happen and who visits.

I hope people will see it's not about cutting them out, but about forging something beautiful and necessary between our child and us. Visits will, therefore be strictly limited and James will play bouncer!

Thirdly, Hyponobirthing has made us consider the matter of baby prenatal bonding. I am pleased to say we have been doing this already quite naturally. This diary is one such example, others being talking/singing to baby, including baby in our conversations, playing music to baby, being conscious of baby, responding to baby's kicks and wiggles. I feel happy to say I've done all these things and more without even thinking about it. James has promised to get his guitar out too and play for her. I'm sure we are headed in the right bonding direction!

24 March 2012

Today has been tiring. I was up at eight this morning to baby-sit little two-year-old Jacie whilst Neil (Jacie's Dad and James's best friend) and James went to pick up our new dining table. It all went really well and I managed to keep Jacie out of trouble until we were sat together calmly on a bench. Prior to sitting on the bench, she had been hurtling round the garden as two-year-olds do. I kept a very steady eye on her in case of incident. Nothing occurred and when she tired herself out I suggested we sit on the bench and watch the rabbits. There didn't seem to be any danger whatsoever.... Then just as I relaxed a little, she simply fell off the bench!

Much tears and hysteria greeted this falling. I felt horrendous and the neighbor hearing the commotion and knowing I have not yet had children, brought me over a toy to try to distract poor screaming Jacie. It didn't work. Well it did for about five minutes, then she must have remembered the fall, and the tears started up again. At which point her mother Natalie magically appeared at our doorstep, having been given a 'heads up' by James who I had texted about my predicament. Mummy was all Jacie needed and she settled down again nicely. Bless her heart though, she did end up with a nasty bruise where she had landed on a metal edge of the rabbit's pen.

I was coping okay, but thank goddess Natalie turned up when she did. This was an interesting taster into toddlers, tantrums and the fact that you simply cannot relax around a child, because as soon as you take your eye off that ball…

After this, we rehomed two of the rabbits. I know I said I wouldn't do this. I really didn't want to. It breaks my heart a little. However, they are going to a good home where people are not pregnant and don't have babies. In the end it is what is best for them. Keeping them may assuage my ego that I am a good rabbit Momma, but I'm honestly struggling to keep them clean and do what needs doing. I'm sure I'll struggle even more when baby arrives. It's the best thing in the long run. I hope they will be very happy with their new Mum.

We still have Lady Madonna rabbit, who, thus far, seems pretty contented with a huge cage to herself. Though my Mum may have found her a new home with chickens and a family who have eight children. So we will see. She may be better off with them being loved and fussed all the time…

I then tidied the garden and sewed new grass. My hips and lower back are sore, which is not helped by an hour in the gym yesterday, but it's been a good day. I had a few moments of emotion. Before lunch I had a true vanity crisis, I went into a state of fear about how I look, but James said all the right things and so I felt better quickly.

Looking forward to a film, Indian takeaway and switching off tonight.

25 March 2012
I dreamt last night that I was giving birth and it was amazing. It didn't hurt and I didn't want it to ever end because it was so perfect. I guess hypnobirthing concepts have infiltrated my subconscious.

Today was my mother-in-law Beverley's 60th Birthday. As she is a twin it was her sister Barbara's birthday too, of course. It was nice to be with James's side of the family. Poppyseed has now been with nearly all our UK family over the past two weeks, between Mike's wedding and this birthday. It's a lovely thought that my little one has consorted with all her people whilst in my belly. Though sadly not my family in Kentucky USA, but as a spiritual person I believe their souls are together now anyway. All of our souls are. We are here and we are elsewhere. Here is complicated, elsewhere is lovely. I hope that the part of us that is elsewhere is readying baby girl up for her arrival, giving her advice, making her strong.

Just over eight weeks and she'll be here. Feeling so contented and as James put it tonight, 'life is good'. We are both so calm right now, life really is the best it has been for a long time.

I've spent the past few years at a computer writing a book or promoting one. None of that matters now, not at all. Life is not in 'becoming' something it is in being, simply being. We can seek a goal all our lives and forget to just be. No wonder we end up stressed out, frazzled and confused about what we want. No wonder so many people have mid-life meltdowns. We forget who we are because we are so busy seeking certificates, esteem, titles, roles and acclaim. We forget that it is perfectly fine to be nothing other than the love in our souls. We forget that underneath the labels, we still exist. Right now, I am very much being. It's better, it's good, and it feels very genuine.

In this moment I'm placing my words in this diary and James is just outside the door training a telescope on the moon. It's lovely. It sounds perhaps silly, but this is a dream come true and I'm so blessed.

28 March 2012

I just brought a towel out to the garden to lie down as it's so hot and then I realized that I don't have the option. I can't lie flat on my back for fear of blocking the flow of the vena cava vein, and I'm so far past lying on my tummy now. Side lying is my only option. For now I'm sitting up cross-legged. That will do. Comfort is rapidly becoming a thing of the past.

The weather has been phenomenal the past few days. It is seriously hot and I love it. I'm not one to shirk a little humidity. My favorite memories are of visiting my family in Kentucky in the summer. It was always so hot we'd suck on ice cubes all day long, and that was part of the charm. Whenever James and I are on hot holidays he tends to sleep through the hottest part of the day either in the shade or in the air-conditioned hotel room. I love to slap on my sun cream and embrace it. Right now, I'm embracing it with a rabbit, cat and book for company. The rabbit and cat are flaking out in the shade. I'm baking.

I'm hoping a bit of sunshine and vitamin D will help because I currently have a cold. I'm amazed that I've gone thirty-two weeks with little but the pregnancy grumps and occasional aching hips and back. Then James got ill with a cold and I've swiftly followed. It's not the worst cold I've ever had, not by a long shot, but I still feel fairly gross. I've taken the day off work so I can do nothing, hence the sun worship. I'm reluctant to take paracetamol as I've gone eight months without it. Last night, essential oils of peppermint and lavender on a tissue was more than sufficient, helping to clear my sinuses and giving relief from a headache. It's my hope a day of rest will winkle it out of my system. I've been munching on fruit too and was tempted to double up on my pregnancy vitamins, but I'm not sure if that's safe, so I won't. Lounging in the sun is my current cure all. I'll let you know how it goes.

30 March 2012
I'm exhausted, still full of a cold and I feel like shit. In spite of that I'm inspired to paint pictures for Poppyseed's nursery and I bought a load of acrylic paint today. I'm feeling creative.

Tonight is Reina's baby shower. I hope I can pull it together a little – things could be so much worse… I just need to shift this foggy headed feeling. I'm going to take a long bath now and then doll myself up. I hope that a little lipstick does the trick.

31 March 2012
I couldn't sleep last night. Coffee at dinner was a bad idea. I ended up sat in the studio with James until nearly 5.30am. I'd say it was frustrating but it was actually incredible. James started playing his most recently written track and Poppyseed went crazy with the kicking. He sat playing one-handed guitar with the other hand on my tummy and we were both amazed by the volume and strength of the movement. Little Miss P particularly responded to the drums and basic guitar sounds. I'm glad she has finally connected with Dad's music. He is going to make the coolest Daddy!

When I did get some rest, I was gifted a vision in my minds

eye. I saw myself in the kitchen and a brown haired little girl ran to me. She had curly pigtails and blue dungarees. She had her own individual little face that was recognizable as tiny pieces of James and me. The best thing about it was her happiness. She was grinning and happy in that way only children can be. What a cutie. What a happy little girl. I'm sure that was a vision of the future and one that makes my heart sing.

It was great to see Roisin and Reina last night. I drove us to the restaurant. Getting back in the car after eating my tummy whacked the steering wheel, where before dinner I had about two inches spare. Clearly dinner made the bump grow rapidly! Alongside my belly bumping, poor Reina couldn't get her seat belt on due to her pregnancy carpal tunnel. We all fell about laughing. Just what I needed…pregnancy-based hysteria. Lovely.

2 April 2012

There is nothing more spiritual than the details of your own life. After years of writing this theory, through pregnancy I am finally living it. I spent a fabulous weekend doing normal practical stuff, creating artworks for Poppyseed's room, cleaning a rabbit's bleeding ear and shopping for house stuff. I've suddenly found so many new hours to the day that I did not know existed. I've watched films, read books, enjoyed baths and done many hypno-birthing meditations; I've planted a whole bunch of seeds in the garden and I've stayed up late bonding with my beautiful husband.

What have I been doing the past few years? Life is here and now. Spirituality is with you whatever you do, but certain things resonate with it better. For me, simply being and indulging in all the simple stuff has been my key. Living peacefully, living simple, living happily though hobbies and sunshine, good food and communication are the way for me. Pregnancy is showing me this. Thank you baby girl, your momma was a little lost but now she is found, Amen.

3 April 2012
For our hypnobirthing homework, James and I are to talk about our fears. I don't really like the word 'fear', but maybe I'm being awkward and trying to avoid the subject. I think mostly our fears revolve around the change we will experience and how that might affect us as a couple, and as individuals.

I know that I've been spoilt as most of my life I've done precisely what I please. That is going to be a hard thing to give up. I know James is worried too that he will neglect his music and end up stuck in a job he hates just to pay our way.

Our 'fears' are not helped by the societal attitude that baby means a stop to life. Women for certain struggle to pursue their own lives, not to mention careers, when a child is young. Many of James's musical friends have fell off the radar when a child came into the picture. Only on Saturday night did someone ask him if the band was finished now he was having a baby. For the record, I doubt that is the case; both he and I are driven people. Baby may slow us up for a while, quite rightly, but it's important we remain true to our other paths in life too, my writing, his music.

I want my baby to see her parents for who they are; Daddy has a guitar strapped to his chest and rhythm in his veins, Mummy writes and does book things and talks of angels, spirits and yes, fairies, why not? I want her to see that dreams are important, and that following a self-made path in life can be done, that following a passion is important, that schooling and structure are not the limit to what can be achieved. I will continue to be me, and James will be he, and her creative old folks, I hope, will inspire Poppyseed.

It is true that in recent years, both our dreams have been adapted. We are in our thirties and prior to being pregnant, we have done a great deal, with some success. Yet neither of us has quite set the world on fire. That's okay though; that was a dream of our twenties that has panned out into something utterly more reasonable. The drive is still in us both, but the need is different. These days I require comfort and a degree of stability. I crave happiness, friends and family. The hunger of crazed ambition was not a healthy place to be and if great things happen, they will do so irrespective of how much I want them to. Life is a tricky old bugger, but I refuse to stop playing because I have a child. Nor will I sacrifice my little girl's happiness for some perverse dream of success. Right now, she is the only success I need.

As for other fears, where do I start? Exhaustion, nappy changing, night feeds, losing my mind (who knows…it does happen). They all rate on my list of concerns, but fears? Nah, fear is not the right word. Fear gives credit and weight and drama to something I am sure I can handle. I can do this thing. No more talk of fear, it is but a word to leap over. From here on I rise only to challenges. In this case, happy baby-shaped challenges.

5 April 2012

Some very random things to report…

Yesterday I had a naked photo shoot. I had booked a bump to baby shoot many moons ago and it finally came around. I spent the night before getting tearful and upset about the state of my maternity underwear. I felt it was all too unflattering to be snapped in. James was adorable and said all the right things, which kind of helped, but I was basically having a pregnancy based 'fat day'. In the end, my bizarre solution was that I would simply do the shoot naked. At least then I'm embracing my 'pregnant' rather than stuffing it into ill-fitting and unflattering garments.

Happily, the photographer was a creative soul who was more than happy to oblige – not in a perverted way. He was an award-winning gent; old enough to be my Grandfather and his wife was his assistant.

We created some really beautiful shots and he even asked if he could use some for his publicity, should I approve them. Confidence now fully restored. Thank you Universe.

On returning home I had an email out of the blue from a production company looking to make a documentary about pregnant women. Specifically, it is looking at couple's different approaches to pregnancy. They had found one of my blogs and seen that I was pregnant. I guess I could be the show's 'spiritual approach'. I'm keen. At first I was not keen. My immediate reaction was 'hell no'. But for some reason I talked myself round rapidly. I spoke to a producer today for nearly an hour and am doubly keen, though nervous. The producer is coming Wednesday, so we will decide then, but for now I'm excited, I think it will be a good thing to do and why the heck not – you only live once. I'll keep you updated, I wouldn't want it to affect James and I in any way, nor would I want it to affect Poppyseed; so that will all be considered carefully.

I did my tarot cards for advice about the documentary. I haven't bothered much with my tarot or any type of guidance card lately. It hasn't felt right. My intuition has been strong, and my intuition has been more than happy to take every day as it is. But I felt this situation would benefit from a little tarot magic. The cards reflect me taking the lead and show James and I being just fine. We have become so tightly bonded over the past few months. I believe that bond would be hard to undo, but then life can unravel so quickly… Appearing in a documentary is not to be taken lightly, though nor is it to be sniffed at.

It's Easter weekend and we are joining the masses in D.I.Y. James wants to finish the nursery and we need to order all the babies furniture, so a practical weekend lies ahead, which is just what we need to distract from photo shoots and documentaries.

I am magnetically attracted to staring at my belly. It's beautiful, it's miraculous, and it's so big and round and perfect. I love it. Little Poppyseed moves around in there and there is nothing but good vibes coming from it.

I dreamt last night that I was in a biker bar in Kentucky. In there I met and befriended a massive Native American guy. He was talking to me and I was listening. He cut off a big lock of his hair I folded it up and put it in my purse. I felt great warmth for him and from him.

Now the reason this is meaningful is that I have always felt a connection to the Native American culture. My family tree tells me that a few grandmas back was a Native American woman native Fanny. So Native American is a little bit in my maternal bloodline. And thus far its influence, so spiritual, trumps other aspects of my ancestral past. Indeed I believe Fanny has visited me once in a spiritual reading coming with books in her hands and offering me them, smiling.

Plus a previous past life regression saw me return to a Native American home and my loving husband who was a much older man. This ex-husband of mine from a previous incarnation has since come forward as a spiritual guide. So maybe last night's dream was a reminder of something deeper from my distant, distant past. That part of me is still with me, through my heritage, my blood and in my soul and indeed it is a part of Poppyseed too.

This morning in celebration of this I listened to some Native American chanting, introducing baby to it. Letting her feel her ancestral and spiritual connections early on. I hope she resonated with it and that her amniotic fluid buzzed with familiarity.

Since yesterday the numbers 1111 and 111 surround me. This happened so much when I wrote my first book and since then it's been 222 and 444 so to be thrust back to the magical, angelic, wondrousness of that innocent 1111 is quite lovely. It tells me I'm guided, I'm protected. It tells me my angels and guides are at hand. Hello Divine Helpers, big loves!

It occurred to me last night that being pregnant is like having an affair with your own body. It's intriguing, educating and right now, I'm in blissed out adoration even in spite of the growing pains...maybe because of them.

Dear Poppyseed,

I want to talk to you about someone who is completely head over heels in love with you, your Dad. Your Daddy has become a new man since you came into our lives. He has spent the past eight months getting the house ready for you. When he speaks of you a light switches on in his eyes. When you kick his hand he grins and looks shy. He is already in awe of you. This past easter weekend he has spent a full four days getting your room ready.

This wasn't an easy task. On Friday he laid the floor. On Saturday he realized that laying the floor had caused a bad leak, which turned into a heating breakdown and a broken downstairs pipe. He had to pull up the newly laid floor and spent all day fixing the various issues. By the end of the day he was tearing his hair out, exhausted and emotional. He just wanted to make it perfect for you. In this madness, I saw a guy totally smitten. In his distress, I saw how determined he is to care for you. You, little girl are blessed to have the father you do, just as he feels so blessed to have you. And I feel blessed to witness what I know you pair will have total, unconditional daddy/daughter love.

Your Dad is going to be your friend, teacher, climbing frame, partner in crime and your guardian. It's going to be something so special and I'm sure this is the start of something incredible. Poppyseed, you and I are so blessed to have your Daddy, he is simply the best.

Yesterday I too had my own realization of how much you

mean to me too. I had been busy all day, when I decided I hadn't felt you kick. Maybe you had and I hadn't noticed, but I truly wasn't sure. I lay around hoping that resting would bring forth some movement. That failed so I downed a pint of cold water hoping to chill you awake – still nothing. It was making me panicky and anxious so I asked your Daddy to say hello, though I didn't tell him why as I didn't want to upset him unnecessarily. In a state of neurotic messiness I went and laid on the bed. Tears were pricking my eyes as I contemplated a stressful trip to the hospital. I asked you to move and let me know you are okay. Finally you relented and my innards were greeted with a volley of kicks and punches. I promptly sobbed my silly eyes out with relief.

My little darling, your Daddy and I are thoroughly in love with you. You've turned us both to emotional jelly. I apologize in advance if we love you too much and worry too hard. I never knew I had such depths of feeling. So go easy on us, because when it comes to you we are irrational, protective and we are certainly wearing rose tinted baby blinkers! You are precious and we are lunatics who adore you. That my baby is never going to change!

See you in six weeks.

Love Momma x

13 April 2012

I've been exhausted these past few days. It's all consuming and as a result I've slowed down. I've not done any exercise as things like climbing the stairs seems exercise enough. James and I had Wednesday off to do our screen test for the pregnancy documentary. It was definitely interesting – all glammed up with nowhere to go – except potentially across a few hundred thousand TV sets in the future! It's Friday today, our involvement is still not definite, but the production folks are coming to film me again on Sunday on my therapy course.

Whilst I'd love to be a part of the documentary I'm also philosophical. I understand we only have six weeks to go before Poppyseed is due and not a huge amount of events to film. So if it doesn't happen I'll be cool and it means I can get on with pregnancy without having to panic about whether or not my make-up/outfit is going to look good on camera. I'll let fate decide this one.

Today I ventured into work for meetings. It was nice to see everyone. Poppyseed was clearly as bored with the meeting as me and squirmed and kicked her way through the several hours. This at least made me more entertained than I might otherwise have been.

I had a midwife appointment yesterday. I complained that I'd had itchy feet the previous night. Unfortunately, as a result, my 'bile function' was brought into question and liver function tests done. I feel it is all a bit hysterical; my feet didn't itch since that one night so I'm not in the least worried. Though yesterday, I was mildly perturbed as if I did have bile build up Poppyseed would likely be born early by Caesarean, which would put paid to the natural hypnobirthing dream, but as long as she is well then I'm happy. Still my liver is fine, I know it.

My course this weekend will be interesting. I get so tired in the afternoon though I am looking forward to it.

17 April 2012

The weekend was great. I was on my therapy course, and on the Sunday I was filmed in class for the potential documentary by a new crew member called Claire. The course, as ever, proved educational and hugely personally informative. Though I was glad when the cameras left so I could relax and scratch my nose without fear of being filmed! It is most exhausting keeping a particular face all day long, in this instance 'the interested student' face, whilst sitting up straight, nodding appropriately and being ultimately overly self-aware.

In class we undertook a past life regression. I was being filmed at this point so did feel a little bit of performance anxiety, but what occurred was stunning to me. I went back to the very first life I encountered when I was writing *The High Heeled Guide to Enlightenment*. It was the life of a nun who had spent her life looking after babies in an orphanage. She had been miserable, old lonely and sick to the back teeth of babies. At the time this shed much light on my current life and why I'd always been reluctant to have babies of my own.

Since that first regression, my mind has changed and children are, of course, very much in my plan. That first visit to the nun, years ago, helped me open myself to having a family. It didn't make me immediately broody, but it helped break down some reluctance. As I revisited this past life the nun had changed from miserable to joyful. Sunshine flooded through her Cathedral windows and I felt that she was so happy that her experience was no longer negatively affecting mine (ours). I guess she is me, but a version of me that is now reconciled with the past and able to move forward in a healthy, happy way. It was delightful to see her again and to know that with the blessing of being pregnant things have come full circle, rectified the old, and started on a new fresh path.

Last night James and I sang a little to Poppyseed, our repertoire of songs needs improvement. Tonight I look forward to laziness and cuddles – we both need it.

18 April 2012

Excuse the excess of information, but I squeezed my nipple and a miniscule drop of water type liquid came out. Wow! I must admit to having been quite intrigued by my nipples for at least the last six months. Not only have they gone so much bigger and darker, but also I've found evidence of what can only be tiny bits of milk. I guess lots of people wouldn't openly admit it, but I have definitely been on 'nipple watch'. As I will continue to be. I'm like a child with a scab and I can't leave them alone!

Speaking of nipples... I wrote an article for *The Huffington Post* that made mention of nipple stroking as a means to inducing labor. Nipple tweeking mimics a baby suckling and in turn promotes oxytocin release. This can then help bring on contractions. Both James and my brother Mike seem quite averse to this comment. Their squeamishness made me laugh. Essentially nipples are for things baby related and I guess guys find it difficult to translate that. Nipples are not playthings, fellas. They are for babies, you guys just borrow them for a while… All I have to say to them is, NIPPLES! NIPPLES! NIPPLES! And here in all its glory is the article!

"Is a painful childbirth all in your head? This is a question that is massively poignant to me, and isn't one that I ask lightly. Seasoned medical professionals and women who have experienced painful births are no doubt baring their teeth. Whilst I don't wish to trample on their experience, I am due to give birth in six weeks and I'm hoping that the title to this piece may be truer than we are currently able to anticipate.

Since becoming pregnant I have explored my options. In doing so I discovered 'Hypnobirthing - The Marie Mongan Method' and my education in natural, empowering birthing began. Whilst I've not yet put the theory to the test, I am already a superfan of the possibilities hypnobirthing holds.

Hypnobirthing starts from the premise that the pain commonly felt in childbirth is not a natural side effect of birth but rather it stems from fear. Women in our highly medicalised society are ingrained to believe that birth is frightening and as they go into labor the feeling is often one of terror. This terror may have been welling in them since childhood when stories of their own birth were recounted, or from the horror tales put to them throughout their life. A pregnant woman is often not reassured by her friends gleeful recitations of tearing, cutting, blood loss, vomiting, labors that last a week and the howling screams coming from a woman in the next room.

This understandable, but culturally driven fear naturally provokes the body's fight, flight or freeze response. All physical energy is directed away from the birthing process and a lifetime of anticipating great pain becomes true, surgery occurs, episiotomies are dosed out, drugs are taken and birth becomes a medical traumatic situation.

Fear ensures that the birthing woman is tense and her body's own natural painkillers, endorphins are therefore blocked. The anxiety in her body causes her to resist what her body wants to do. The hubbub that surrounds this in the hospital; machines, midwifes, invasive examinations simply causes her to slip further into a state of panic. It is no surprise that so many of our gals are left begging for the numbing sensation of whatever drug happens to be closest.

Birth is taken from mum and placed in the hands of professionals and all she is left with is another horror story to pass on. Of course some women may have a medical need for medical intervention, but midwife led centers such as The Farm in Tennessee run by Ina May Gaskin, have proven that surgical interference could occur in as little as 1% of births.

Indeed many other cultures experience childbirth as an empowering, straightforward, intense rite of passage for women. They don't understand what all of our fuss is about. Yet physiologically we are identical. It's seems to me that our sophisticated society has moved childbirth beyond itself. In medicalising birth and creating fear, we have disempowered women to the incredible power of their own bodies.

Hypnobirthing aims to place the power for birthing back in the hands of the parents. The formula is such a simple one. It involves removing the fear, relaxing, going inward and guess what... trusting our bodies. Yes actually trusting that women have birthed for thousands of years, many in a time or land without chemical or surgical interference, and they have done so quite nicely.

As a hypnobirthing devotee, I'm currently learning to trust my body and my baby to do what comes ever so natural. I believe I've conquered my fears of childbirth, and I am looking forward to the whole process. I know - how peculiar! As is my husband who having attended the hypnobirth classes with me could not argue with the fabulous logic of it all.

I'm not suggesting it won't be a challenge, or that it will totally pain free, but visualizing that the intensity of natural birth will be a wondrous occurrence. I am placing trust in my uterine muscles to do what they are meant to do effectively. I will handle challenging moments with a dose of deep relaxation, total faith, and if it comes to it, some nipple stroking from my nearest and dearest. Yes nipple stroking and other gentle touch techniques are said to flood the body with oxytocin, enabling an easier birth. Many may balk, but I'd rather get a little bit fruity in the delivery room than lose my marbles or physical control to chemical interference.

In a few weeks time I hope to report that my baby was brought into this world the old fashioned way. It's my mission to relax and go deeply inside the physical me, prompted by my spiritual inclination for gentleness, peace and all things natural. This is the first soulful gift I can give my little girl. A birth that is not only anticipated with excitement and big huge love, but delivered with it too."

You know you are very, very pregnant when pajamas and

comfort clothing hang where your skinny jeans and fancy dresses used to be. The fancy/skinny stuff is all relegated far, far away, which is better for my mental state and self-esteem. It is important that everything in reaching distance fits to feel good. I really don't need to be experimenting with whether my pre-pregnancy wardrobe fits right now. It is surprising what doesn't fit. Things I would have thought had plenty of room, or that I considered baggy prior to pregnancy are no longer as baggy as I believed. It's not pleasant to see the buttons of one's favorite baggy shirt inches from doing up, or a T-shirt I considered to be long, now riding up over my belly button. Indulging in dress up is a one-way track to feeling bad. Instead I've assured that everything I can reach fits loose and lovely.

It's been occurring to me today that my focus on hypnobirthing, whilst fabulous, is also problematic. In being so zoned in on the birth, I'm forgetting the more important aspect of what precisely is being born. Not only that, but in some respects hypnobirthing is aimed at the avoidance of fear/pain, but in actively avoiding them am I not constantly being reminded that they are a possibility? So as of today, I will take my hypnobirthing lightly. Once baby is here, none of what has happened will matter one jot. So whether I have a blissful birth is, in some respects, irrelevant. Hypnobirthing sets a good background for baby entering the world and it is important to me. But it is not something I want to take over. I want to use the tools I am given, but the main goal here is to birth a beautiful baby. One way or another, my little Poppyseed is popping out and the process will soon be as relevant as last week's newspaper.

I'm going to focus on that end result a little more. The idea of Poppyseed being here is the thing that really wipes out my fears. So with that in mind, and a dose of hypnobirthing relaxation, I should be set for the trip of my lifetime.

The book based on this diary was contracted today – what a blessing. Life is good, things are coming together in ways I never contemplated, wished for or could ever have guessed. Between books, TV documentaries and my blogs being read by more people my hard work is paying off. I guess the Universe has some plans for me. I guess I'll do my 'birth' breathing and go with the flow. It seems my body and my life know what to do, I just need to turn up and facilitate where I can! To think all the time I've tried to be in control and gotten nowhere... Lesson learned.

Dear Poppyseed,
Hello my little one. The time of our meeting is creeping up slowly. I wish I could keep you safe inside me forever, but at the same time I am so excited to see your little face, hold you, play with your perfect fingers. I have high hopes for us little darling. I know you already and I know our souls are friends. I know that through thick and thin you are my blood and a soul mate. I adore you little lady. I love you.

Mummy is planning a beautiful Blessingway ceremony. Lots of people have 'baby showers' where the Mum-to-be is given loads of gifts. I don't want that for us. I want your way to be blessed, and for the women I love to gather together to give us love and support. What I want from people is blessings, power and good vibes not baskets of baby goop. It almost feels cheekier asking people for their blessing, for their love. Love and blessings are harder to give for many than simply handing over a gift certificate or pack of baby vests. I guess I'm being awkward, asking so much from people. But I know these people, you will know these people, and I know they care, so blessings, candles and beads (to be strung together and worn in our labor) are the way forward. All our girlfriends will hold you and me in love and support and this will grant us much strength on the day of your birth. I can't wait for the Blessingway. I have a feeling it will be a beautiful day.

Love, Momma

20 April 2012

The documentary filming is now official. The crew is going to be around a lot more often, so I will give them names, they are Claire and Donovan. They are filming James's gig tomorrow, filming me Wednesday, both of us Thursday and again next Saturday for the Blessingway Ceremony. It's very exciting. I hope to get lots of filming out of the way now so that I get some time to myself towards my due date. I'm sure it will work out as it's supposed to…

I saw Reina last night, she's due in six days and looks stunning, in full bloom. It was lovely to chat about our plans for hanging out when both our bubbas are here. We are both praying for a good warm summer so we can play outside with our little ones. Though not too warm; so there's no pressure to strip down too much before our bodies get back to some semblance of normality.

We both talked about how much we appreciate our pre-pregnancy bodies. Whilst we've both had good pregnancies, there's something about those final aches and pains that has made us grateful for the total freedom of movement that we had before.

On another fantastic note, one of Poppyseed's future playmates is starting to show his or her self. My friend Gaynor has been having contractions for four days poor woman! I hope that baby gets itself into the world sharpish and relieves its poor momma.

It seems I'm infiltrating other people's dreams. Two people have confessed to having dreamt about my pregnancy. Delilah, a friend from Soul Café, dreamt I was heavily pregnant whilst another girl I know, confessed I was pregnant in a field, and was in labor, so she shipped me off to hospital. Following which she dreamt that James told all the guys how much he fancied me! Bravo I say, good dream.

Strangely, or should I say non-coincidentally, we studied dreams at the weekend on my therapy course. The upshot being that in dream interpretation the things we dream of represent ourselves. So it is flattering that people are equating me with a part of themselves, a maternal part, no doubt. I could do with remembering a few of my dreams, I could do with the entertainment, but my crazy dreams seem to have ceased for the time being. *Desperate Housewives* (my latest addiction) is becoming rather staid, a good dreaming session would be most welcome.

James showed me a video application of himself looking like an old person on his phone. I couldn't stop crying. It was only a silly phone app, but it broke me. He looked so sad and lonely as an old fella. I think perhaps today I'm destined to be over sensitive. Hopefully not too much though, because we are going out baby shopping! Having been given so much stuff and having bought all the big bits and pieces it's finally time to make some little purchases. I'm not a huge fan of shopping, but in this instance I can't wait. Little girl sundresses ahoy! Though James seems to think baby can live in an, "I (heart) Ozzy Osbourne" baby vest, I have assured him that my one and only little lady deserves some frills.

Oh, I've come over all pink and girly!

23 April 2012

Yesterday was lovely. What was supposed to be a partially relaxing Sunday turned into organizing the baby's nursery. We chose green as the main accessory color, which looked gorgeous with the plain white walls. Being a nature girl, green sits perfectly with the environment I want my baby in. Plus it is a soothing, healing color in terms of spirituality. So I'm very happy with that choice. The nursery is looking very classy, and very cute. It's all seeming so real and exciting.

Today, I woke feeling a real sense of happiness. It occurred to me I have everything I need and want. Given Miss P arriving perfect and healthy, life is good. I was a little overwhelmed by my positive feelings; I felt them not just towards my life, but also towards friends, family and acquaintances. It was blissful. This was followed by hot flushes and a good half hour of queasiness. I'm pretty sure the hot flushes were unrelated to the happiness, but both are, no doubt, a result of hormones!

Had a work meeting that proved to be fun. Spent time with some lovely colleagues, made more wonderful with the sure knowledge that I only have three working days left till I'm on maternity leave. Whilst my maternity leave will be spattered with some writing work (I hope to catch up on some articles before baby comes) and filming, it's still something to look forward to. This is very much the plan presuming that baby doesn't come early, as everyone is intent on warning me right now.

Something happened today that was a little bit heartbreaking. I witnessed a friend of mine torn apart by her teen daughter. A teen daughter who until a few months ago, was a bright shining star but who has now fallen into the clutches of first love in the form of a dodgy boyfriend. I hope and pray it resolves itself and the girl comes to her senses. First love is such a powerful feeling and many of us have lost out heads to it. When it happens you truly believe in it, even when it comes in a package that is far from the stereotypical prince charming.

My first love was a decent guy but I lost myself within that relationship completely. It took a good long while to rediscover who I was following that. Like I said the guy was a nice chap with education, prospects, decent upbringing, he was by no means dodgy but… Love can be a bind and it can be blinding. It's one of the most powerful, uplifting and sometimes destructive forces we allow into our lives. That said, we all have a path, we all get to where we are going via a litany of mistakes and errors.

This past weekend on my therapy course I heard a roomful of similar stories about relationships. We had a session of talking about our lives, and every person had been scarred by one or more relationships in the past, particularly those first relationships when we were younger, more naïve, more ready to throw our hearts and heads in without thinking. Not one of the stories was pretty, but each person had stood up and overcome every ugliness they had endured.

So I hope and pray that my friend's daughter sees the light and saves herself sooner rather than later. Seeing her mother's love and worry is, of course, not lost on me right now. Whilst I hope Poppyseed never does similar, she could well do and I, as a soon-to-be mother feel my friend's pain more poignantly than I would have done eight months ago. One thing I'm learning from all this, is that whilst first love is intoxicating, fascinating, addictive and romantic love can be beautiful; parental love is a whole new animal. I can feel already that it is unconditional, powerful and I fear utterly relentless.

Feeling tired today. Four weeks and two days to go! As of tonight the cats are barred from the bedroom at night. Molly cat will not be happy, and I'm feeling it pretty hard too as she is my little hot water bottle. I bought her a new cat bed and hope that will suffice. It's best to start now than have cats that resent the child thrust upon them. Cats are resilient, so am I. We can do this!

24 April 2012

Totally failed at the first meow. Poor little Molly has such a plaintive emotional cry, so I relented and let her in, one last night together, with James's blessing. I will try again tonight, this must be done.

I am now definitely feeling eight months pregnant. My brain-power is rapidly vanishing. I feel okay whilst in the comfort zone of my house but as soon as I leave it, and have to embark on a voyage of several steps, weird aches and pains reveal themselves. When I stand up, the weight seems to shift into my pelvis and it's less than comfortable. I didn't sleep well last night and this afternoon I walked out onto the road into the path of a car that I swear came from nowhere. Alongside this, I've been a bit needy and wholly expect James to drop everything to entertain me. James, however, has been making the baby's nursery look even more gorgeous so entertainment is sparse.

Whilst a few weeks ago, TV was my comfort I'm now bored of it. The gym isn't really an option so the highlight of my day thus far was planting tomato seeds. Also, I had a psychological test from a real life, suited and booted psychologist – to make sure I'm sufficiently sane to be filmed for the TV documentary. These two events were so much fun in my mundane schedule that I tried to have a little dance. I'm a wiggly hip/tummy dancer, this didn't work and it turned into more of a hand jive. Still I enjoyed myself and am very much looking forward to having a wigglier dance with little Poppyseed on my hip once she's here.

In other news, I've cooked a super-healthy dinner involving butternut squash, spinach and leek. James is soon to be by my side providing an entertainment function. And Molly cat is able to use ladders – which is rare for a cat I hear. She is perhaps feeling the onset of change and has taken herself up to the attic a number of times, via the ladders. Poor thing can get up, but not down.

Tomorrow is a day of filming and I have a few things lined up to be caught on camera. I have Mia my Doula coming and I'm having a sound bath along with Reina. A sound bath involves Sarah from the Sacred Voice coming along to play all manner of awesome hippy style instruments such as rattles, crystal bowls and singing bowls. She will also chant and do magical two-tone style singing. This sound bath is a form of sound therapy, I experienced it previously and it is delicious and blissful. I'm looking forward to that. Plus it's Reina's due date tomorrow so it could be interesting to see what the vibrations bring.

Have been a bit slack on the hypnobirthing practice but I do feel that my mind is in the right place. I'm looking at birth in all new holistic and yet also realistic ways. Whatever happens I get a baby at the end. That is most definitely the way to see things.

25 April 2012

Four weeks to go! Can't say the pressure isn't getting to me a bit... James is still working so hard on the house and I'm anxious we won't spend any time together till baby pops out. I know, in part, I'm being irrational but I'm missing him so much as he devotes himself to D.I.Y. His projects have got super intense as he tries to free himself up to be with me for the last few weeks. But to me it seems never ending, if it's not a leak that needs fixing, it's a pile of wires that needs sorting. In the meantime, my emotional wires are backfiring, I really miss him. I really just want to be with him and for him not to be wielding a screwdriver/hammer/paint brush.

On Saturday night, I sat on the Studio couch with him till late and its only because I can't sleep because he is not with me. Pathetic I know. As he is being fairly nocturnal, it's messing my sleeping habits up. But I'd rather be with him for half an hour at 1am than not at all. I need the house stuff to be finished because it's trashing my otherwise relaxed and Zen state of mind. I need my man back.

Dear Poppyseed,
It's your Grandma Becky's (my Mummy) birthday today. I'll never forget that her mum (your Great Grandma) once told me that she is always reminded of G'ma Becky's birth by yellow tulips, as when she was born the yellow tulips were blooming. I'll have to make efforts to notice what is popping from the ground when you pop out of me. It's a beautiful way to remember a person. Whenever I see yellow tulips I think of my Mummy now. I was born in September, so I guess when you see trees starting to turn color to rich autumnal reds and yellows, you can think of me!

You've been kicking and squirming so much lately and I've taken to stroking your body parts as they individually stick out from my belly. I hope you like it, though if you could avoid the downwards kicking towards my bladder I'd be grateful! Love to you little baby belle.

26 April 2012
Yesterday was a full day of filming. Loads of people were in and out of the house and the crew; Claire and Donovan, oversaw the lot. Happily, Claire and Donovan are really personable and easy to chat to, otherwise this filming lark would be a real bind. But they are sweethearts, they make it easy, it's a little bit like having friends around. Friends with cameras! Friends who ask you to repeat what you said, but to say it more concisely for the camera. I really need to learn not to waffle. I'm very good at long answers, the shorter one's seem to be harder to come by. I guess it's a good job I have a waffling outlet through my books. But on film, no waffling allowed.

I had a great day and very much enjoyed being the centre of attention. I won't lie, as a child I loved to act. I was forever putting on plays for the parents and forcing my brothers to be my acting buddies. There is a part of me that still feels more than happy in the limelight. A few years ago I rejected the world of acting after starring in a local play. That play nearly killed me, as did a brief stint of modeling. But this real life documentary stuff, this is ok, I like this.

Whilst I enjoyed the day, it took a difficult turn in the evening when James started to express a wish not to be involved any more. This started as a whimper and transformed into a roar. He did not enjoy the filming as much as I did. He felt stressed by coming home from work to a camera in his face. It was, to be fair to him, very awkward... He did not have the chance to warm up as I did. He literally opened the door to filming in his face. Not a great start for the guy who likes to have five minutes man time downloading the day before even talking to me! Now that he has nearly finished decorating, he is suddenly feeling he has to fit into some kind of TV role. He is not the natural that I clearly am! He can get on a stage with a guitar and be a showoff…sorry I mean showman. But cameras in the living room are a different matter.

We talked until really late about this and the feeling I got was that we should drop out. He didn't say this; he knows how much I want to go ahead. But seeing him so stressed about it, when previously we were both so excited about the baby, was distressing for me. I didn't sleep well at all. All I could think was that he was only doing it for me, and that we may regret it. One of my provisos on this whole thing was that it should not affect our life together. And it was doing... So after a terrible night tossing and turning first thing in the morning, I telephoned the producers to drop out.

At that point in time, all I could see was the need to protect us from the stress and Poppyseed from being over-shadowed. I endured several calls to various TV people from the production company. They really didn't want to let me go. The phone calls were not easy. They didn't pressure me to continue, well no, I'm lying, they kind of did pressure me…in a nice, personable way. This sent me back to bed with my head spinning and my heart a little bit breaking. I felt torn between what I wanted, what the TV people wanted and what I was worried may happen to my life should we go ahead. I went back to bed exhausted. Somewhere in the dreams that followed an answer came to me. I dreamt that I needed to compromise and that I should go ahead with the filming, but, by myself. The dream was quite bizarre (as ever), there was a pink baby carrier, and Gary Barlow from Take That encouraged me to go ahead with the documentary, but without James. Gary was very convincing. I woke up feeling much happier; I felt that the dream was a direct message from my inner knowing and one that made sense. It cut through the crap and struck a good balance. Filming alone meant that James was unaffected and I could follow my heart.

I rang up Ruth at the production company and we negotiated. They were willing to make changes for me so that James was not involved. Although I know that they hoped he would be, even if just a little bit. She also offered to cut down the number of dates we have for filming and work round me due to me being so far ahead in my pregnancy. It's nice to be wanted and to also connect with the producer Ruth, who, like me, is spiritually inclined. This made me feel more assured that I would not be shown in a crazy light. She is coming to see me tomorrow, and hopefully that will cement this new decision for me.

James was happy with the new arrangement and despite the drama of it all, I'm glad it happened. I'm sorry people were messed around, but I guess sometimes drama finds itself right where you aren't expecting it. In this instance, it cleared things up for James and whilst it was an emotional roller coaster I'm glad we found a way through, rather than enduring a relationship implosion some way down the line!

The thing is, though, that now the pressure is off James, he's suddenly not wholly averse to being involved. Whereas before he felt huge pressure he is suddenly happy to get involved as and when the right opportunity arises.

In other lessons related to this, I think it's important James and I keep a good distance in what we do. Our private life is precious, but when we try to get involved in each other's work things go wrong. I'll always adore his music, feedback to him, and be the first person to hear it, but I wouldn't go on stage with him or ask to conduct the band's haircuts. Same goes for him, he encourages me and is interested in my writing, but he doesn't feel right being involved on an active level. So we made a pact, he does his thing, I do mine, we adore and love the other and their work and then we come home and are the James and Alice that exist behind closed doors.

27 April 2012

Ruth came to see us. She spoke to both James and I. We are now very much backtracked. Filming will go ahead and James will be involved. Now he has been reassured, and he is calling the shots on what he is filmed doing, he feels better. I believe fear was struck into his heart when it was previously suggested that they wanted to film us, in the woods, James with a guitar in hand, me doing hippy incense wafting in the background. He felt this didn't represent him, so he went diva. I don't blame him. It doesn't represent him or us. But it was just an idea, and he realizes he now has the power to say No. He used that power, and he liked how it felt enough to continue with the documentary, with the proviso that we don't do hippy wood dancing, and we are only filmed doing things we would actually do!

29 April 2012

Yesterday was remarkable. It was Poppyseed's and my Blessingway ceremony and it was beautiful. We started off the day early just pottering and preparing. First to arrive were the film crew whilst I was still in my pajamas, followed by Roisin, Hayley, Reina, Mum and Mum-in-Law Bev. There was much preparation, hair doings and chatter going on. Much of this was filmed, but like me, it seems my friends are naturals.

After twelve everyone else started to arrive. Some naughty folk brought gifts, which was kind. But of course unnecessary as Blessingways are about celebration rather than commercialism. That said gifts are, of course, welcome and all go toward helping us prepare for the new arrival.

Soon my little living room was full of female bodies and two camera folks so we got started. I had only just sourced a blessing to read myself. It only occurred to me the night before that I should read something too! I then searched for two hours on the Internet only for James to remind me about an amazing children's poem we had heard read on a film the night before. So I went to bed and he found the words for me. This was what I read out to start us off. Having searched for my own blessing I knew how hard it was and I had a newfound respect for everyone who had done that for me. It occurred to me that buying a gift would have been a far easier option!

It was deeply emotional as we worked around the room and I was overwhelmed with love from my beautiful girlies. At the start of each reading the reader lit a candle and at the end they shook the rattle. In between this, little baby Jacie, our youngest guest, took a liking to the rattle and shook it randomly, which had a charm of its own and was no doubt her own way of offering a blessing.

My friends and family made me feel so loved, warm and secure that they would be here for Miss P (and me) in the future. Though it was my Mum who brought the house down as she sobbed her way through one of the most emotional moments of my life. The poem she chose to read was *'I Carry Your Heart in Mine'* by EE Cummings. It was stunning. Afterwards I gave her a big hug and felt very blessed. When I turned round, it was clear to see that Mum's speech had affected everyone, for all I could see was a sea of tissues, running eyes and nose blowing. Adorable.

At the end, I collected a bead from everyone and my step-mum Aileen strung them together for me. The beads represent everyone's spirit and I will wear them in labor to connect me to people and give me strength. Just as when I go into labor I will contact everyone who was present at the Blessingway and ask them to re-light the candles in our honor, whilst sending us power and good wishes.

After the ceremony, we all ate the food everyone had brought, we chatted and gossiped and a party atmosphere reigned. Now the other thing that happened which truly made the day special was that two little announcements were made to me in top secret. Two good friends of mine both confided in me (separately from each other) that they too are pregnant! How very perfect.

So many of my best friends are becoming mommas. All these girls have been my buddies, my confidants, my drinking partners and we have over the past ten years shared so many memories, so many fabulous times and at my Blessingway so many of us were sat there with new life in our bellies. Not just the physical new life of our children, but the new life of our own. Pregnancy is a real inner trip, a chance to reflect and rediscover who you are. It is life changing even before baby comes along, this new internal life is set to merge with baby's new physical life and again transformation will occur.

Today James and I went to visit our birthing centre. It was great to sit in the room where Poppyseed may be born and see the reality start to unfold. As we sat and chatted to the midwife, little

Miss P moved and wriggled constantly. I think she knew…maybe she was wondering why we were there early and if anything was expected of her? The midwives at the centre are well clued up and informed about hypnobirthing. This will make life easier. I feel so excited and whilst I want baby to stay inside a little while longer, I'm also really keen to get to that room again, but next time I'll leave with a little bundle and less of a bump!

After visiting the birthing centre, we went food shopping. Up till now, I've been doing food shopping alone. But I was so grateful for a hand. Even simple things like bending into the trolley to retrieve items has become an intense activity. So assistance was sorely needed. We now have all kinds of food in the freezer waiting to be slammed in the oven for easy meals after baby arrives. We also have a whole load of stuff for our hospital bag, so much that you'd think we were packing for a fun road trip rather than a potentially long birthing. Though best to prepare for what you want and why the heck can't the birth be a fun road trip? It is after all taking us to a whole new place… I have also ordered a selection of essential oils as recommended by the midwife at the birthing centre; sage, lavender and frankincense, we are so nearly ready.

1 May 2012

Today is my first day of freedom! Well it's the first day of maternity leave. Last night I had a lovely dinner with workmates. They had so kindly clubbed together and bought me a sling for baby, I can't wait to use it! It felt peculiar to know that the day job is wrapped up for the time being. Of course my work is never done and I've already written an article this morning amongst other bits and pieces.

Have spent some time fussing Molly cat. Last night saw Molly piteously crying at the bedroom door to be let in. Today sees me super stalking her out of guilt. When I can be bothered to get dressed I'm nipping out to buy her a cat bed to go on my desk, the last one I bought her has Jimi cat squatting in it. I love that cat so much and it's important she feels safe and not pushed out.

In Molly's defense after some small time meowing at the door she gave up and slept all night on the bed I made her in the bathroom, she didn't even try and follow me back on one of my many nighttime trips to the toilet. So there is hope that little Miss Molly Anna Tallulah Moo (her full name) will soon accept the new set up.

I'm still sleeping really well. The bump is not preventing that, thank goddess. Though the past two nights I've woken with odd cramps in my pelvis and stomach/uterus. I guess these are Braxton Hicks practice contractions as they feel a little like period cramps. They don't stop me sleeping, and they don't seem to happen in the day, nor are they getting any worse. Maybe my body is gearing up for a nighttime start to birthing. In my imagination, labor should always begin at night, the dead of night. To me, lunchtime seems an odd time for labor to begin, mid-afternoon stranger still. But I guess either is possible. Though for me, the dark of night is my preference.

This weekend is a super moon. I'm hoping that this does not bring on labor. I need a few more weeks. Just a couple would be fine. My request is for a few more lazy mornings, a bit more hypnobirthing meditation practice and some more filming and writing time. That would be lovely, that is my intention, two or three more weeks to do what I need... That is my request to the universe.

Yesterday a pregnant friend texted me to say that her husband had been made redundant; this is a complete and total bummer. Life can be a real cruel place to be sometimes, from happiness to hell in one fell swoop.

That said, my experience of pregnancy, as a spiritual life-altering event, is that this kind of thing is liable to happen. You get pregnant then the cosmos slaps you right down. As awful as this may seem, it's a relevant challenge. It's a divine way of letting you know that everything changes now. You are no longer boss and you'd better make suitable changes to your life to pull you up to the level required of you by your unborn child.

Perhaps having a child is a unique circumstance within which divine energies can knock you into shape. I know since James and I got pregnant, we have been thrown many a hurdle and we have had no choice but to leap and leap and leap. As a result I'm different, James is different, we are better. We are becoming less selfish; we are more loving, giving and forgiving. Little things carry more weight; we are so much more grateful for friends and family. Life is a whole different reality and it's because of those dark dingy hurdles we had to cross. So I hope and pray that my friend surmounts hers too.

2nd May 2012.

Today was lovely, my mum-in-law Bev came round to help with cleaning and we chatted lots about babies, James, filming, what to wear… It's great to know what a hands-on Nana she plans to be. It's definitely going to help give me space to do my thing. Having missed having Grandparents in the local vicinity when I grew up, I am so grateful that Poppyseed will have Nana Bev living so close by, as well as two other sets of grandparents living an hour or so away.

James had an emotional moment in a pub today as we waited for dinner to arrive. A beautiful song came on and he drifted off in his mind. I suddenly notice his eyes looked a little watery and I asked if he was okay. He tried to claim he was, until that little bit of water grew in volume and splashed down his cheek. Apparently this keeps happening and it's totally baby related. He loves that little Miss so much. When we got home I showed him a video I had watched yesterday of a gorgeous baby having a bath, and yes the effect was the same. Rock 'n' Roll James again welled up and had a little moment. I've logged this emotional display in my memory box, to be revisited during labor. Knowing that labor is giving him such a lovely gift will make any discomfort or pain worthwhile.

When we were chatting over dinner James made a good point about birth. He said that the fear around it was a bit like being worried you would be hit round the head with a frying pan at some unknown time. Whilst you can mentally prepare for this inevitability, when it eventually comes it's still going to knock you sideways. Hypnobirthing and spiritual la la aside, he had a point. I'd better get ready for fried eggs 'cos that frying pan is headed my way.

4 May 2012

I am being filmed as I write this. Claire and Donovan have been here since yesterday. We are doing a writing sequence and so here I am doing it and writing about it. Weird! So yesterday James and I were interviewed on camera, some interviews on our own, some together. James has jumped back into filming with gusto. As soon as the pressure was off he decided that he wanted to be involved. At first he wanted only to do a few music related scenes, but it was not long before he threw himself back in fully. Once he felt he was back in control, he was good with it all.

James and I had fun together filming, when being observed like that; you cannot help but notice the nature of your own self and each other. I was acutely aware of how we interacted with each other, as well as noticing our personalities. I noted so much that I normally take for granted when there is no camera tailing me. I remembered that James is hilarious and saw that he is clearly quite proud of me. I hope he realized too that I'm proud of him. It is definitely a one off experience this random filming. A strange mirror to our life together, I must say.

5 May 2012

Thank god there is no filming today. Lovely as the production team are, it's still an exhausting and disrupting process. I felt that I was 'being' myself for the whole time yesterday, which is far harder work than simply being myself. If that makes sense? After two days of 'being me' for the cameras, I'm depleted. Last night I felt detached from my own reality and myself. I couldn't get my mind wrapped around having this baby and it wasn't pleasant.

One good night's sleep later, and I'm back on form. I pottered around this morning and cleaned the house. I went to the optician, went shopping and carried the bags back rather than drive. It was a perfect day of little things and nothingness. I've missed these small things in two days of filming. I'm doing some more filming Tuesday, but it's not at home, so may not have the same draining affect. Really looking forward to making dinner tonight and doing very little afterward. I'm sleeping brilliantly too, so that is such a blessing given my crazy schedule. Well, crazy for a woman who is eight and a half months pregnant anyway!

As part of the filming we met up with my Doula, Mia Scotland again. She was also the teacher at my hypnobirthing class. She asked if we would be having Vitamin K for baby. I said I'd research it. Today my *The Mother* magazine arrived with a feature story on Vitamin K splashed across the front - perfect timing. And in answer to her question, I can now say a resounding, though slightly on the fence "unlikely". Given the ideal birth that I anticipate I don't believe Vitamin K will be necessary.

This morning I saw a blackbird in the garden. There are never birds in our garden. I've not seen one for years due to the cats. I know a sign when I see one and blackbirds represent transformation. Transformation is, of course, something unavoidable right now.

As I write this, I'm sat in the bedroom whilst James empties wardrobes and boxes into bags for charity shops, this is just one small example of our current transformation. I have thus far bagged up nearly all my handbags and a pair of boots that have remained unworn for nine years. Our wardrobes are thoroughly transformed.

✡

7 May 2012

Having a lovely bank holiday weekend. Yesterday we went for an Indian buffet with Neil, Natalie and their gorgeous girls Lainey and Jacie. Afterwards they came back to ours for a few hours and we all slobbed out on the sofas watching family TV. I'm feeling very full.

Today James and I are going to the local tropical bird land. It's something I've been trying to get him to do for years. It seems today he has finally succumbed. This weekend of normalness has been much needed, it's so important to touch base with simple things like house cleaning, seeing friends, eating too much and having a cuddle with cats / kids.

It's great not to indulge ones vanity too much, as TV filming tends to encourage. When the cameras are here, I can't help but study my hair, nails and make-up in minute detail. Being with a few friends relaxing means I can go easy on the beautifying regime.

Natalie, who has had one unfortunately painful and traumatic natural childbirth, told me that she couldn't see how hypnobirthing will ever work. Whilst I want to disagree with her, it's hard, because only she knows what she went through. I've never done it. What do I know?

In hypnobirthing I have a theory that I love, but I love it because it suits me, not because I've tried and tested it. So whilst her opinion riles the bit of me that wants to believe in pain free birth, it is also impossible to not acknowledge and appreciate her honesty.

In hypnobirthing we are advised to ignore the negative stories, and I try...but there are so many... It's culturally normal for women to shock others with their awful, painful, and traumatic, near death birthing stories. Surely all these women can't be wrong? Although that's what hypnobirthing suggests. It suggests we are buying into the cultural belief that birth is painful. When really, according to hypnobirthing, if you relax and breathe correctly it's not painful at all. Again I say, surely all these Women can't be wrong? But then I see the hypnobirthing films of peaceful, tranquil, beautiful births. I have to hold out for that. I have to.

Perhaps unsurprisingly, I had an intense night of anxiety dreams about birth last night. I can't remember the details. Right now I'm going to write down my fears and my hopes about birth and burn them in the garden. It's a letter to the universe hopefully setting intent for what I do and do not want and need.

Here is what I'm burning:

I release fear of birth being painful, frustrating or scary.
I embrace birth as a powerful empowering act.
I am excited to meet baby.
I call upon the universe, divine power of nature, my own inner divinity to assist and nurture my birthing. I ask to be kept safe and happy throughout birth and after. I trust and have faith in my body. This experience will be beautiful and soul inspiring. My baby will be well, as will I and James.
I am not afraid.
I am empowered.

I am in control of relaxing and releasing at every stage.

I am going to kick ass and freaking love it.

Thank you universe for this gift. Together we will do this thing well.

All my love.

Alice

9 May 2012

Got loads of errands done today, which felt worthy and pleasing. Even filling the car with silly expensive petrol felt strangely fabulous. I now have a tank full of petrol that will doubtless last till well after baby is born as I have nowhere to be and nothing to do. Getting petrol is a pet hate of mine, it's such a hassle. So time off doing it is time well spent.

Yesterday was a photo shoot for this book's promotion. Scott Gilbert, a good friend and wonderful photographer came over from Cambridge to take the shots. Though he almost didn't as the studio we had booked was a no-go. After arriving at the studio Scott discovered that a bunch of their lights were broken. The owner firstly advised us to "make-do". On second thoughts he said his wife would pick up new bulbs. By this point my intuition was well set against the place. James suggested using a local music studio that houses big airy, light rooms, so we headed over there and got some beautiful shots. This was all filmed for the documentary, and whilst I went at my posing full throttle, I cringe to think of myself and my naked bump being viewed by thousands. I felt quite vulnerable. At the same time, I enjoyed the day, had a laugh with Scott and found out later that a famous band had been in the room next door. Damn, I could have got them to sing to Poppyseed!

James came along for the end of the shoot and to indulge some banter with Scott. Afterward we headed home and I did nothing all night except watch my stories on TV. At the minute, I have a *Breaking Bad* marathon going on, but am also taken by *Weeds*. TV is my good friend again. James buzzed around doing man things and it was generally a lovely night.

10 May 2012

Today I've had a variety of pelvic aches and pains. I don't feel that Poppyseed has dropped into place yet, so I guess it s a mixture of her squirming and my body preparing itself. Some of the pains have been quite sharp, but tickly at the same time, which is why I think the culprit may be Miss P and her wriggling.

James's mum has made a prediction of 10th as the date of birth. She said if not the tenth, then the twelfth. She is keeping her options open! The twelfth is not ideal as James has a gig that may be filmed as part of the pregnancy documentary. I want him to have that opportunity so I hope she is wrong.

A psychic friend of mine Deb, came up with the number twelve. So I'm choosing to interpret this as in twelve days, from, now, which leads us to the 21st. The 21st would be preferable. I also have my therapy course this weekend and I'd be sad to miss it, being as it's played a vital role in the pregnancy.

So Poppyseed, if you are somehow feeling this message, can you give me at least another week, ideally please arrive on the 21st, 22nd or 23rd . I'll keep you warm and safe till then darling. Hope that's a fair deal. Love you little lady!

11 May 2012

I am shattered after a busy day filming. It was not a great night's sleep last night, either. I feel like I'm in a negotiation with something I can't control, constantly bargaining with baby bump about when it's convenient for her to arrive. Now, for example, is a bad time as I'm so tired. Tomorrow or Sunday is not great either as James and I have plans. After that I'd love a couple of lazy days. As you can see, I'm bargaining with this and it's silly, but I keep doing it, as if I can make a genuine difference.

I know I don't get to decide, but maybe spiritually I hold some sway? If all energy and life is connected, which I believe it is, I may well get some influence? Either way, I resolve to be happy because even an inconvenient or inappropriate birthing time would still result in the best thing ever.

This all pales in comparison though to some news I got today. One of my dear friends who confided in me that she was pregnant at my Blessingway has been bleeding, having cramps and now it seems has lost her baby. I'm so sad for her. I know so many people this has happened to and I just feel terrible for them all. I don't care how early on a pregnancy is, it makes no difference... Once you know you are pregnant you are in love. So to lose that loved child, even at such an early stage is a massive devastation. I really feel for her, and send her so much love. So much love.

12 May 2012
No baby as yet. I'm thinking that Bev's psychic powers are a little off in her prediction for today's birthing. I'm super exhausted and I feel massive too. Several times in the last few days I've had people gasp at my size. If I was feeling less confident I could take this personally, but realistically they are not wrong. I am massive. The mass is mainly on my belly, but I know the old muffin top is suffering too, whilst my face, I think is looking a tad bloated and sleepy.

Tonight, James is playing a gig in London. I've negotiated with Poppyseed Bump not to come out, though if she does I would hope James has sufficient time to dash home.

I forgot to say! Reina had her baby, a little boy. His name is Pepe Shay and I met him today. What a sweet little lump of gorgeousness he is. Reina seemed to be doing good too, despite having an induction followed by a caesarean when Pepe was found to be breach. I was so excited to meet him and I can't wait to see him and my girl grow up as friends.

Reina told me that labor, as far as she experienced it, doesn't hurt. I was, of course, overjoyed to hear that. She said it is not an actual pain, but rather an all-encompassing intensity. I needed to hear that, it certainly sounds preferable, challenging but preferable. It backs up my hypnobirthing learning's and I like it.

Dear Poppyseed,
Whilst you aren't born yet, I want you to know that the fields are abundant with bright yellow rapeseed blossoms. Tree blossom is falling but springing up from the ground are bluebells and buttercups. Summer is coming and bees have started to appear. For the last few weeks there has been a glut of ladybirds in our garden. My tomato plants (second batch) have failed to grow but my peas look promising. The grass is growing swiftly, spattered with dandelions and whilst it has rained for several weeks, the sun is shining bright today.

I believe you'll be with us soon. You have been moving about far more than usual. You have gone from little pixie like shadow in my tummy to definite little human. A little human made up of your Dad and I, grown in the greenhouse of my belly. Watered with love.

Love you little girl, see you soon!

Mama.

14 May 2012
Sleep is so important for me right now, it helps me keep perspective. Yesterday my tiredness left me feeling anxious, but after a good night's sleep I'm ever so excited. Miss P is on her way soon and I don't care what the birth brings as long as it yields her up safe and sound. Stitches heal and pain is temporary. Family is forever. I feel I've been in a transient phase, not yet ready to let go of my bump but suddenly I feel heady.

Whilst I'd love another week of maternity, I'm far more ready now. Yesterday, the blackbird visited again and she stayed in the garden even though both of the cats were there. She is heralding our transformation.

15 May 2012
I'm shattered. I slept so well but I'm utterly pooped. Yesterday Mum and Karen took me for lunch, and then kindly bought us our shopping and loads of baby bits. They too are gearing up to be Grandmas! At night James and I just rested. Yet today I feel so drained. Having a pajama day, and then going to the cinema tonight.

My problem is that there is always a list buzzing round my head of things I could/should be doing. It's hard to ignore it when I'm on limited time. But none of it is essential, even my book writing or my course homework can all wait.

So, for today, I've cleaned the kitchen and typed up our birth plan. That's enough now I think. I'll watch some of my stories on the TV and have a bath. If I feel more awake later then I'll do my course homework at the least. Tomorrow is a filming day so I need to keep myself rested, well and truly. I've requested that the film crew go easy on me and so we are planning a two-hour break at lunch, which I know I'll need.

James keeps suggesting I go for a jog and eat a curry, bless him! I've told him a resounding: No, but...maybe at the weekend. Well maybe the curry, not the jog! Though I am sure there are more interesting ways of induction we could explore...off to cinema with James now. Possibly our last, none babysitter required date. My nipples are tingling, that's not happened for months, intriguing.

16 May 2012
Last night we went to the cinema, came home after lovely time, and then before I went to bed I absolutely lost the plot. I could not stop crying, I was apportioning the blame all over the place, to being tired, to James, to TV filming. The next day I felt fine. Exhaustion is getting the better of me now, I think I'm not doing much, but maybe the small stuff I do is too much? I was crying over absolutely nothing. I've also been suffering strange aches and pains. Essentially my baby is getting ready for birth and my mind has short-circuited into a full on meltdown.

James was absolutely gorgeous to me. He was so sympathetic and kind, it really helped me gain perspective and go to sleep happy. Prior to pregnancy such outbursts may have frustrated him. But pregnancy has taught him how to handle an emotional woman and he does it so well. No more does he snap at me to pull myself together, instead I have a caring, sympathetic, understanding fella who speaks golden words of wondrousness that send my malaise reeling and helps me to feel so loved. After his kindness I slept so well.

Today has been filming all day, probably the last lot of filming before baby arrives. I'm tired, but as ever believing that all things happen for a reason, even tiring filming days.

I was supposed to have a break during filming but a flat tyre, the same tyre that I had replaced last week, scuppered this. So frustrating. But if Donovan hadn't noticed I'd still be driving round on a dangerous flat, so again all things happen for a reason. Plus Donovan and Claire, who I am feeling are almost a part of the family now as they are here so often and we are becoming increasingly chummy, escorted me to a garage to get it sorted out. They are a handy pair; every pregnant woman should have her own personal camera crew for such emergencies!

It's been strange having the crew around. I haven't written a lot about them, because usually after they have left I am far too tired. But I have to say they are a welcome addition to the end of my pregnancy. They are friendly, helpful, sweet and generally lovely. Plus they are hanging out with a whole bunch of other pregnant people so they often have great tips and advice. Considering the fact that filming could be very stressful now, they make it easier.

I had my midwife appointment today. This confirmed that baby is engaged in my pelvis, not wholly, but she is definitely on the way, which explains the aches and pain.

Did some filming with James today, packing hospital bags, calling taxis to get prices to go to the birthing centre should I go into labor at an inconvenient time. The production team do keep us on the straight and narrow. Had they not been in our lives I think we'd be far less organized. It was them who suggested we might want to consider how we would get to the birth centre. Intriguing how all things, including documentary filming, offers blessings.

18 May 2012

I am finding the limitations of my body irritating. I feel great round the house but then as soon as I step foot out of it, the aches kick in. I can come down my own stairs, but a few steps in the local supermarket and I am seizing up. It's all good fun though; pregnancy is an interesting ride, including the aches and pains.

I'm lucky in that having had a healthy body all my life, mere aches and pains are a novelty. Such aches and pains are a beautiful sign of my imminent arrival.

The only side effect I do not love is the touch of boredom an aching body brings about. I don't feel like I want to be venturing out on my own in case of a labor type situation occurring. So it's the sofa, the TV, the computer, the kindle, a bath and me. Managed a touch of gardening today but it was fairly gentle and rather halfhearted.

Just been on a supermarket trip with James. Got all dressed up with a splash of make-up. What a treat! An hour or so later I'm back on the sofa in my slobby clothes. I'm now the proud owner of a breast pump too. My work today is done. James', however, is not. He is still seriously nesting. Today he is sawing bits off the bed to make it lower. I'm not sure why. I think he doesn't know how to stop… I'll let him get on with it. I am so past caring about spending 'couple' time together. We have had our fair share of that. He is a little busy poppa bird, feathering the nest.

A couple of days ago, I really felt baby was on the way sooner rather than later. Today I don't feel that so much. She is due now in five days and whilst my guess is Monday (today is Friday), I'm not sure any more. It's the kind of thing I hope to get some kind of psychic sign about, but nothing is forthcoming. It's weird to know that labor could crack off at any old time.

I'd love for it to happen in the early hours of the morning, so I've had some sleep, but the rest of the world is still dozing. I'd love to sit and have a cup of tea with James as the sun comes up, knowing what is about to happen. I'd love that little perfect moment of time before we have to do anything or tell anyone. That is my wish, but realistically it could be any day, any time, it could be now or thirty minutes from now, or it could be another two weeks yet. It's a strange kind of limbo, a limbo that I want to last so I can indulge my freedom, and a limbo that I want to end so that the future is now. So I guess I have no choice and no real options, I simply sit and dwell and be.

Physically, I'm feeling proud of myself. I was advised that for a healthy pregnancy I should put on 2 stone, no more, no less. I weighed myself yesterday and found I had put on precisely that! I am hugely happy about that. All by accident too, exercising, eating what I fancy, but not going crazy.

I have a whole new perception of my body, she is not something to be feared, purified or starved, she is good to me, and she is not wayward or bemusing as I once believed. I actually know her better than I realized; I must remember how amazing she is when it comes time to burn away the extra fat, and I will trust her to help me do it right. Well done my body, you are a star!

19 May 2012

Strangely I don't feel pregnant any more. I feel instead that I am expecting. It's like cooking I suppose. For nine months I've been cooking up my child. Every move she or I made was vital to the perfect outcome. But now I feel she is cooked. She is simply on simmer. Her movements are slower and the oven is turned right down. We are both just waiting for the mystery moment when the buzzer goes off and the final product is delivered with a ping.

So in spite of my lumbering, waddling presence, I don't feel pregnant, I feel transitory, I feel ready. I am burgeoning. Baby and I have taken this journey, this inner meeting as far as it can go. The next phase looms and I can almost feel it, but until that cooker is finished I'm still officially pregnant.

Materially I believe we have everything we need. Today we brought the pram home and already I've had to wrestle the cats out of it several times. The house is well stocked with all things for baby, to the point I don't think we are missing anything. The

Grandma's have been incredible in helping to get lots of baby necessities. Whilst gifts and hand me down from friends and family have made up the rest, and I guess there will be more of that to come.

James has stocked up on rock and roll baby vests, we have Jimi Hendrix, AC/DC, Ozzy Osbourne and a Queen one. We have sufficient toys for a newborn. The nursery is perfect, the house is perfect, and James and I are perfect. I won't wish this perfect simmering time away, in its own gentle way it is perfect.

Physically I can't stop eating. Eating and peeing. I'm trying to have small snacks. They satisfy me for a while, and then I get ferociously hungry again. I can't ignore the feeling, it is so strong and so I've eaten quite a lot. Maybe baby and body are storing up some energy for labor, who knows, but I've been one hungry mother. Between eating, I've been visiting the toilet more. The bump has definitely dropped and so a little special someone is leaving less room for my bladder. I sat at my desk for an hour or two earlier working on my writing. My back and pelvis were horribly uncomfortable and I felt drained afterwards. Right now I'm back to the incessant TV watching and book reading.

In relation to hypnobirthing, I have been doing a little homework. I tend to listen to the meditations in the morning as James leaves the house and they send me back to sleep. I'm feeling good. Hypnobirthing has given me the key to it all. This key is knowing that there is no need to feel fear and relaxation is everything. Breathing and visualization are all I can do to make that real. I am embracing a belief in my body's ability to get the job done, naturally and without relief. I'm not scared, I'm anxious, but mainly because I don't know what to expect from any of it. I have stage nerves, but am sure that I'll perform well anyway. Birth is always the unknown, as is life, but what I do know is I control my experience, how my mind reacts is vital, what I allow my body to do and not do is my choice. Birth is in my court and I'm going to serve it up well.

21 May 2012
Well it's about nine at night and no baby yet. It seems my theory for today being 'the day' is out the window unless I go into labor now and produce Poppyseed before 12pm, stranger things have happened! My pendulum had predicted the 22nd so I guess tomorrow could be the day. The 23rd is the due date as dosed out by my health care providers. After that it's anyone's guess!

I didn't do a lot today, slept in, tidied the house, and hung around feeling a little lost. I'm not very good at relaxing. That said I'm back in front of the TV now watching episode after episode of American drama. I seem to have a current penchant for drug dealing crime dramas. As a result I've learned a lot about the Drug Enforcement Agency and the fact that married couples need not testify against one another in the US. Who said TV rots the brain? I'm all set if James and I move to the States and embark on our own drug empire.

Felt like a caged animal today until I went and met my friend Annie for a decaf Chai Latte. Annie is a woman from work who I hit it off with recently. It was just what I needed to pull me out of my enforced relaxation doldrums. Came home to James clearing up the garden in the sun. It looked stunning out there. It's no Kew Gardens, but it's pretty, and it's ours. So looking forward to Poppyseed and I spending many a sunny moment together as I do the weeding and she watches the bees.

Whilst writing this, I just had a weird sensation in my body that felt like it stemmed from down below. It was not unpleasant, but it set my nerves on edge even though it was very faint. It has not repeated itself and it may be nothing or it may be something. I don't feel there is much more waiting to be done. And yet I can't imagine it at all, I really can't.

22 May 2012
Today is gloriously sunny. After weeks of overcast skies and rain, today is sweltering. I had a cup of tea in the garden first thing and it was hot already. I love it. I'd rather be too hot, it's delicious. James and I are making the most of it and are going to have a barbecue when he is home from work. I went for a walk to get supplies and was overjoyed when a lady asked me when I was due and I got to tell her it was tomorrow! The highlights of my day are far simpler than they used to be.

This afternoon I'm going to sow more tomatoes and eat fruit. That's it. God bless the sun, it truly helps me relax. After days of grudging attempts to chill out, under the sun's rays it is suddenly so easy. Indeed I hope Miss Poppyseed may give me a day or two more pregnancy so that I can thoroughly take advantage. Today was the day of birth as predicted by my pendulum, but I never have been too convinced by pendulums. My tarots are better trusted and they do not suggest that today is the day. So, I'll go with them and hope for time to bask under the big yellow sky ball.

...Have done all my sun worshipping and tomato planting, loved it. The sun is one powerful feel-good maker. I am suddenly so excited. Everyone who I know who was pregnant at the same time as me have now had their babies, it's me next, I'm excited beyond belief. I'm so ripe and ready.

The fact Poppyseed has almost reached her due date means I've savored every last minute of the forty weeks. From now on, there is nothing to miss out on, but there is so much to look forward to. The whole situation has shifted. Before I wanted to keep her in and ensure I got everything out of pregnancy. Now I can look forward to meeting her. I'm not impatient, I'm unafraid, and I'm in massive anticipation.

Dear Poppyseed,
Today is your due date and you woke me up wriggling around. I feel closer than ever to you as we prepare for your arrival. My pelvis and hips are aching, but beyond that I feel fabulous. I'm so excited to meet you. I can feel your spirit starting to move forward. I can envisage having you in our home and whilst I'm not sure who you are or what you will look like, I know you on a whole other mysterious level. You are in our lives just as I'm sure you were planned to be. I don't mean plans made by Dad and I, I mean soul level plans… When I came to the earth you came with me. You and I are written in the stars. We were always going to happen. It was always going to be you.

Several years' back when I had a super broody phase, I named you Dakota and I knew you'd be here one day. At that point I missed you dearly, I needed you. Since then, your Dad and I have rejuvenated our love, and our life, and now I don't need you. I am whole in myself, I am satisfied in my life, I am truly happy in my skin. So, no I don't need you now, instead I love you, I want you, I miss you. I am ready to be the parent you deserve, precisely because there is no need involved. There is only purity. The nature of life has taken this course as it was meant to. My life has re-jigged itself so that your arrival coincides with the best version of your Daddy and I that I've ever known. You will add to our little life party and together we will live and love and grow.

We simply can't wait to get you involved. We want to build you up, show you the sights, and help you to be happy and well rounded. That is our mission, little lady.

Don't you worry too much about arriving today – what do Doctors know anyway? But when you are ready, know this, we, little lady, are very ready for you.

Love always, Mum

23 May 2012
I'm sat in the boiling sun and its only ten in the morning. It's my due date. I'm not feeling it. I had thought baby might be early, but now I don't feel any kind of rush. I don't feel much like making predictions either. I have no attachment to any date, it is a mystery to me.

I have done my forty weeks of pregnancy and that was my dream. I didn't want to be early of that by even a few days, so I am content that I happily enjoyed the lot. It's been a marvelous pregnancy too. James remarked yesterday how straight forward and undramatic it had been, which I hope has passed on to baby, giving her an easy growing period full of calm and peace. Having flicked through the pages of this diary, I see many of the entries are ones where I might be moaning or overemotional. Yet I have escaped serious physical side effects and my ups and downs have not been so bad, not really.

Physically. I've been so lucky. Even now I am not swollen, constipated, bloated or suffering in ways so many other pregnant women do. I'm doing alright. I've had aches and pains, not big ones, little ones. It's been a pure joy, any mood swings I've had have been easier to dismiss due to my overwhelming happiness at simply being pregnant. A good nights sleep has often sorted them out. Besides in any nine-month period some mood swings should be expected, pregnant or otherwise. In general I'm just happy. Pregnancy has been enlightenment, a gift, I've been philosophical, I've reviewed my personality and I've come out shining.

Relationship-wise we have gone from a place of trouble and attempting to overcome a period of misery to being in a place where we have successfully overcome everything. We are solid. I am more in love now than at any point in the past ten years and in that love I feel deep peace and safety. Peace, safety and a massive crush on my husband who in his newfound happiness looks hot as hell. God, he is gorgeous. I keep sneaking peaks at him and look forward to a little more one-on-one time when there is no longer a third party in the room with us! Though with co-sleeping on the agenda that may be a while in the future…

Spiritually, I've changed too. More than ever I see spirit in everything and no longer feel a need to seek it. Spirit is a pleasure, but it's not why I'm here. I can honor my spirituality really and only through my life, and so it is life I embrace but always with a soulfulness in my heart, intuition in mind and one corner of my eye looking out for coincidences, miracles and signs that might help pass time on earth in a more fruitful way. I have faith and that is enough. It's in my heart, but my heart is full of baby too and right now she comes first.

So today is my due date and I feel calm, serene, and happy. These past forty weeks have changed my life for the better and forever. Whatever happens next I'll never forget this time, this precious, treasured miracle portion of my life. It's quite simply been the best of the best.

24 May 2012

Yesterday was another filming day and I expected it to be a couple of hours maximum. In the end it was 3.30 till 9.30, not to mention the time prior to that getting ready and prepared. At the end of a fun day I felt utterly shattered, painfully tired. I went to bed in absolute terror I may go into labor, but happily I did not. Hopefully, I'll get today to recover before Miss P makes herself felt.

During filming we went along to a local country park and sat on the same bench we had sat at the day we found out we were pregnant. That felt bizarre, being in the same place nine months on. It was a nice place to reflect and see how things had come full circle. On the way back to the car we came across a mummy swan with one little baby. The cygnet was adorable and I took the liberty of naming it after our baby. Now there just needs to be a baby to name…

The sun is still shining like crazy and its hot and humid, which may have added to my exhaustion yesterday. Am sat in the garden now taking in some rays and sweating profusely. I may be forced to retreat inside shortly; this is not the time to get a suntan. Everything is harder right now. Physically I'm definitely feeling the effects of being very pregnant.

My step-grandfather died yesterday. He's been ill on and off for years, mainly on though. I remember Dad saying maybe two years ago that he was probably going to die then. He did well staying around, although perhaps it's not been the greatest of times, in and out of hospital so often. He leaves his wife of sixty-two years, which is terribly sad.

What I know of bereaved women, however, is that they may tend to surprise everyone with a hardcore, impressive existence. My Grandma Grist has flourished in her own ways since Grandpa passed. We didn't expect that. Women are survivors. So I hope Dorothy survives Eric too and experiences some peace and happiness for however long she wishes.

I wonder, perhaps, if Poppyseed has allowed Eric his chance to leave before taking over as the new centre of attention, if so I am very proud of her little soul. Maybe as she is incoming, and he is outgoing, they can meet up briefly to swap family notes. As for Eric, the notes on him were that he was a gentle bear of a man. A gentle, loving bear. He fed us too much chocolate and took me to his Masonic Ladies Evening as a budding young woman.

I was bought a fancy velour black dress from the catalogue and loved the night being spoiled by Masonic types. It was my first ever fancy outfit event and I felt so glamorous and grown up. Yes, Eric was a man to be remembered.

My midwife appointment today uncovered that baby has not yet engaged her head in my pelvis. Though last week she had apparently engaged. Confusing? I have spent time since the appointment adopting all manner of positions, over chairs and across birthing balls trying to help her get her head down. It may well be that I could go into labor and contractions would force her head down anyway. If I can help her out I will, as the less time spent in labor the better. Maybe baby hasn't engaged as I keep asking her not to come yet? Maybe she has simply respected my wishes. On that note, I formally state that after tonight's sleep, my little Miss Poppyseed is welcome anytime.

25 May 2012
A poppy has opened up in the garden. I hope that this is a sign.

I had horrid dreams last night of gross infidelity and girls from my old school. Not pleasant at all. On the way home from a pedicure I drove past a lorry named Poppy and a car with a poppy attached to the front. Poppies everywhere today. Maybe my Poppyseed is getting ready to bloom.

26 May 2012
Three days overdue. Tired, nauseous and grumpy. Slept in till 10.30 but feel like I must have sweated half my amniotic fluid out in the night.

The sun is still shining beautifully but I feel like a swollen beached whale, I'm enjoying it less. None of my bras fit well, they are all too small. My boobs feel swollen and huge. I bought some stretchy sports bras to tide me over, but they are too small also. There is no point getting decent bras right now as following birth my breasts are going to change radically again…

Invited friends for a barbeque to try and distract us. Whilst purchasing food at the supermarket I was forced to listen to the checkout girl telling me all about how childbirth is the worst pain ever, several times over. She then proceeded to tell me how spoilt and annoying her kids are. Apparently though, it's all worthwhile...

Part of me wanted to stop her in her tracks and tell her all about hypnobirthing, part of me wanted to scream at her to shut up, another part smiled and nodded politely. Seriously who tells a heavily pregnant woman, past her due date, how much pain she is about to suffer? Who does that? I think I may be feeling a tad irritable.

There was no point in challenging her, it's her experience, she meant well and she really was being friendly. If she'd realized how much she was affecting me I'm sure she'd have felt devastated, I let it go. Though a part of me grizzled all the way home. All the way home to find our neighbor had all the doors and windows open and her music blaring across the neighborhood. This is the very reason I would not want a home birth.

I need to go get grounded. I bought a bunch of disabled and exhausted looking strawberry plants. It's my mission to give them a new lease of life. Must go do that now, but not before I find my earphones and turn my music up loud.

27 May 2012
The hot days drag on relentlessly. I feel very much as if I've stepped outside of time. A few days ago we expected a baby any minute. I've stopped expecting. I am floating in an alternate world of pregnancy sweat. It's not tedious, I asked for extra time but I didn't really expect to be given it. Now that I have no real time frame I have naught but hot weather, bedtimes and moments to fill.

Last night we filled moments with Neil, Natalie, Laney and Jacie and another barbeque. We bought a paddling pool for the kids and the evening flew by. We ate, they drank, and we were all merry. The kids ran around naked, it was cute. This morning I have worked several hours on the garden losing blood and sweat but as yet no amniotic fluid.

Little Poppyseed is bobbing around in my belly, perfectly content it seems. Tried sex this morning as an induction attempt, but I suspect our baby is sufficiently decided on her birth date and no old wives tale will alter that. I think I'll look back at this time as a moment outside of itself, a moment unlike any other. Days and days of glorious, hot summer. I have a big belly so huge now it is disabling and a strange peacefulness settled around me.

We don't even talk baby right now. We talked ourselves out by due date and so now there is a verbal absence. Realistically, she will be here soon one way or another. But my hopes and expectations are not geared towards guessing when. We are living second to second. My nails are studded up with garden dirt. My thoughts are turning to finishing a painting I started and reading my new book.

Dear Poppyseed
What is going on with you little love? No hurry darling, we are ready when you decide. Until then, your Dad and I will whittle away our last remaining childless days in a calm and peaceful manner. We are looking forward to meeting you - happily we are past impatience and planning. Maybe you are like us, you do things on impulse. When the impulse takes you to come earthside, then I will be delighted to make your acquaintance.

Sending you big love and cuddles to tide you over till birth time.

Love, Mummy.

28 May 2012

After a week of bright blue skies and hotness beyond what Britain is accustomed to, the sky is suddenly full of clouds. I feel it may rain soon; maybe this natural change will prompt an internal flood in me too.

Today I've visited a dear friend who broke up with her boyfriend at the weekend. I lost myself in her troubles for a while and enjoyed her company, enjoyed being there for her. I also had the opportunity to complete an article I had started for a National magazine last week. Perhaps Poppyseed is kindly allowing me to do such things before she limits my attention.

In the time since she has been expected, I have actually made some massive inroads with my writing and I've also had some fabulous time with friends, family and to myself. Miss P really has been generous. I feel I have caught up on so much, as well as laid some new paths for the future. I'm on top of things and it is liberating and exciting. As I write this, the first few drops of rain are falling. Maybe I paid too much attention to my Shakespeare in school, but could this be a pathetic fallacy, rain representing an inner cleansing? Baby is moving more all of a sudden. I feel her partying a little lower down my pelvis. The rain is really falling now. I'm going to go out and get wet…

…I'm sat here now with droplets glimmering on my skin. A little of Mother Nature's juice may be what I need right now.

Before the rain started, I had been reading a spiritual magazine and was prompted to choose a symbol from an array on the page. The symbol I chose apparently meant I needed to complete something in my life. No kidding; a whole new person needs completing!

I've just been for a lovely walk with James at the pretty lakes near our house. On the way to the lakes, I saw a clairvoyant and therapy centre that I'd never noticed before. We stopped on the way home and apparently they were talking about a pregnant woman when my belly appeared at the window. A man came out and invited me in. It seems like I've stumbled across a great little therapy centre, one that has been in place for three years and so is well established. Could this be a perfect place for me to practice my therapies, meditation and tarot in the future maybe? I think it seems that Poppyseed really is helping set her mummy's future up for her. For every day she has been late, I have been gifted opportunity.

Her being late has allowed inroads, big and small. I've become a regular writer on a few big websites and magazines plus now I've found a local snug base to work from if I decide to take that route. I'm so blessed, Poppyseed is my baby angel. Every day extra has been a gift. Thank you Miss P.

29 May 2012
Today Poppyseed's gift of time is for her Dad. He has the day off work and a new guitar arriving. It was delivered nice and early and now he is getting the chance to play with it. Having spent nine months making the house look pretty he really deserves this time out!

Baby is feeling lower today. Apparently my pubic bone is bulging out. I definitely feel more going on down low. So maybe it's nearly time.

30 May 2012
Still pregnant... Had to make a hard decision today on whether to have a membrane sweep or not. It is a slightly invasive procedure where the midwife tries to separate the membranes

around the cervix with her fingers. It's more effective than eating curry, less effective than chemical induction. Part of me was very tempted to go ahead and have it, because it could possibly bring my girlie out, but in other respects it just felt wrong. The key to my pregnancy and indeed birthing and hypnobirthing is trusting my body. The NHS would rather I trust them but I feel strongly that if baby was meant to be here, she would be.

I do feel that she is making her way to me and I don't feel right pushing that quite yet. My intuition didn't sit right with it and so I refused the sweep today (Tuesday). I have, however, booked to have a sweep on Friday should she not arrive by then. So baby has a couple of days to move her butt, otherwise my choices become limited and interventions may have to start. The reason I will have a sweep Friday is because if I don't and baby still doesn't come, then I'm booked for chemical induction on the following Monday. At that point I will be twelve days overdue. According to my doula, twelve days is nothing. I agree. Baby is not officially considered to be overdue till fourteen days after her due date. So I think perhaps I will refuse the induction at twelve days, but I'm hoping it won't get that far. I desperately don't want to be induced.

In comparison to induction a sweep is the far, far lesser of the two evils. So we have two days left to get this thing done totally naturally, and five days till drugs get brought into the equation. I trust that this is enough time.

I did myself a reading prior to making a decision on the membrane sweep using guidance cards. The cards I got were Rebirth and Power. Rebirth was all about gestation being complete and the hardest time coming just before birth, but also strongly spoke of trusting and having faith. Whereas Power was about not seeing power as good or bad, black and white but simply learning to tap into my own universal power. With all that in mind I'm looking forward to a day to myself where I can meditate and chill out and do whatever comes naturally to help provoke my little baba out with naught being used except a momma's love. I've turned my computer off and I'm going barefoot and fancy free from now on. All my energy is for baby and birth and I can't risk getting myself busy and wasting energy. This is a full throttle redirection of all energy inward.

31 May 2012

Booking in for an induction yesterday has made me realize just how much I want the natural birth we have planned. I know life doesn't always go to plan, but oh my gosh, do I want this. As such, I'm making all efforts to make it happen. If it doesn't, then I guess no one can say I didn't try. Last night and this morning I prayed on the subject. I sent my intention out to the universe and I hope it was heard.

Before I fell asleep, I went really deeply inward to my baby. I explained to her what might happen and I asked her to work with me so that together we can set our intention to avoid chemicals and get things moving. As I sent her these thoughts I stroked my belly and she reacted throughout with little wiggles and kicks.

All night long I dreamt that I was taking baby to see loads of different wise men that were all advising her about birth. I don't remember the details but I felt it was helpful. This morning I woke really early and feel she is perhaps a little lower and I was definitely feeling more aches and pains.

I'm now sat watching TV and have just given my belly a rub with Clary Sage oil mixed with a carrier, I rubbed a little of this into my feet too and am going to have a bath soon with a few drops mixed in with that. Clary Sage is supposed to help bring on contractions…

I am hoping to book for reflexology this morning. I'm seeing my Doula, Mia, this afternoon. In the meantime, all I'm thinking is baby, baby, baby, birth, birth, birth.

...I've been for reflexology, which was bliss, and I've been to visit my friend Gaynor and her new baby Maisie. Somewhere in this time frame I've had a change of attitude. Before I felt a little desperate, a little stuck on a natural birth. Now I feel inclined only toward a birth. I must be comfortable with the fact that life does not always go to plan.

Had a telephone consultation with Mia as I couldn't bear to drive all the way to her. She did a 'hypnotic induction' for me. Apparently they can be very effective. I will wait and see.

Mia pointed out that in accepting induction on Monday I am robbing baby of two precious days of her growth. Ninety-five percent of babies come on their own by two weeks after their due date. So, if I was in the five percent that doesn't come within the two weeks, then I guess that induction is a route I'll have to consider. But two days are a lot to steal from a child who is not ready, two days is nothing to us, but a great deal for baby's development. Particularly when that child is having a very normal healthy pregnancy. Nothing has changed in that respect, I don't feel we should rush her. Clearly the medical professionals feel differently. I trust Poppyseed can do this of her own free will in the next week and make induction a redundant point.

That said, I am booked for a sweep tomorrow, a lovely wise lady told me today that a sweep is a physical violation. I see where she is coming from but I disagree, if I've given my permission, and I'm happy with it I really don't see it that way. This whole panic to get baby out by 'term plus twelve' days is a violation. The thought of induction is a violation. So a sweep is the only power I have to counter all these other violations. I know I could go super alternative and refuse to play along with the medical agenda, but it's my first baby. I daren't. My Mum would kill me!

Besides, sweeps often don't work. They don't force baby to come, but they do encourage. Which makes me believe that if baby doesn't want to move, then she won't, and no harm done. So a sweep I can agree to, it's okay with me, I don't know what else to do. But an induction, I hate to agree to, not before Poppyseed has had a chance to ripen as she wishes or requires. I will refuse to be induced on Monday. I will submit to monitoring or whatever is needed, but I need to buy my Poppyseed time.

None of this is to my plan. I believed Poppyseed would be here before the due date. So now I'm contemplating things I didn't think I would have to. Somewhere along the line I have to give up and trust my intuition, and whilst I've taken on board all the facts and opinions, it is essentially down to what I feel is right. Induction doesn't feel good, I don't want to do it before I absolutely have to. I think two weeks extra, a full two weeks past due date, is not asking a lot. After all my clamoring for a natural birth, I think that extra two days of growth is wholly reasonable. I feel baby is so nearly ready anyway. For the next week I surrender to her and to my body, after that I may consider surrendering to the medical folk, but not before baby has been given her full notice period.

A lovely thing happened today. I went to get money from the cash machine for the reflexology. When I got back in the car, the radio announced that the song "*Small Bump*" by Ed. Sheeran was up next. James and I listened to this song so much when we were first pregnant. Hearing it now made me realize how very far we have come. It also reminded me what this time is all about. What really matters is that lovely small bump. The one who has stolen my heart.

The tarot card I got for today is Full Moon – completion. When I was first pregnant the full moon card came up all the time. So this seems meaningful. When I read the meaning it specifically said that gestation was done. Any period between gestation and revelation may be tedious (as it is) but is vital to the big reveal. I look forward to that big reveal and I trust it will come as naturally as possible.

1 June 2012
Looks like little Poppyseed will be a June baby then. Last night James and I went for a walk and I had Braxton Hicks style tightening the whole time. It was relentless. I was hugely uncomfortable in my pelvis, bladder and, yes, my bowels. Had to stop and pee in a bush as I thought I might have had a drastic accident. I also had some period style cramping. I awoke after a good night's sleep…still pregnant.

I have now officially moved the induction date until fourteen days after the due date. I really wouldn't want to do it then either, but they are insistent. The past few days have been so stressful trying to balance the information from the medical folk with the info from my Doula, Mia which is far more liberal and in agreement with my own intuition. As a Libran, I find such balancing acts essential. I can't come down too heavily on either side as both sides have convincing arguments. I am pulled more strongly to avoidance of the medical interventions being offered, unless such interventions are totally necessary.

The problem with induction is that in undergoing it, you are placing a healthy pregnancy under a medical cosh. One intervention often leads to another… Then the trauma of birth that I wish to avoid is played out tenfold. It is my deepest desire that baby finds herself ripe and ready before any of this becomes a reality.

…Today I have agreed to have a sweep. I've felt so torn about this decision. I truly believe that whilst natural is best, we are a tooled up society and someone having a feel around my cervix is tame in comparison to the other option. Christ I've succumbed to far, far worse in my family planning needs over the years. Whilst there is a medical cosh with induction, I also feel that there is a natural birthing gang who may tell me I'm doing wrong by having a sweep at all. But it feels fine to me; it feels like another possibly effective technique that's worth a try. I guess I'm a bit desperate and desperate times call for desperate measures.

It also seems baby and body can freely ignore should they choose to. If a sweep helps avoid a chemical induction, then I'm all for it. Just as my body ignored all the other options that I have tried, reflexology, hypnotic induction, walking, curry, sex, aromatherapy, meditation... My body still has a choice about this one. If a membrane sweep helps keep me far from an induction team, then all the better.

The thing I really need to remember is that baby will be born when the time is right. I believe that all things happen for a reason and so however this plays out, it is meant to be…simple.

James wrote some music today. He asked me to write some lyrics. To inspire myself I took a guidance card that was all about breathing properly. This struck a chord as hypnobirthing too is all about breathing. On top of that I have been stressing about induction, and I feel perhaps my breathing has been insufficient and far too shallow.

So this poem/lyrics seemed to fall out of me. Along with a new very natural plan… From here on in, until baby is birthed and born, all I intend to do is breathe. To breathe well and deep and long. I've started already in the past half hour; I feel nice, very calm. Baby is moving and I'm getting more twinges. So that is that. Breathing is all I intend to do. No more crazy curries, no more trips to get rubbed and poked or anything, just baby, breath and me. The perfect ménage a trois.

Breathing your soul into beating
Deep and slow and low and long
Come to me in all your needing,
Into the light, my little one.

Your first breath yet to take

Hollowed out in your lungs
Time to step toward my healing
Breathe until you feel reborn.

Power of lung meets power of heart
Flesh and emotions torn apart
Find me through my breathing song
Together forever, my Little One.

...As it happens, the midwife could not do a sweep. Baby's head is still too high up and my cervix is not dilated enough. Damn. I'm lost with regard to all this medical stuff. I'm mildly glad because I wasn't overly keen on the sweep in the first place, having previously refused one. So now I'm back to breathing and relaxing. I will also visualize baby getting her head further down and coming naturally.

The film crew was here today and they are such sweeties, it was a nice distraction. A few weeks ago we thought they had such a short time to film me for. But baby has granted them an extension. I wonder what the story of my birth will be? Today is Friday and I have till Wednesday before I am the two weeks overdue and the talk of induction gets serious. This gives Poppyseed five days to remove herself willfully. I have been asked to go into hospital on Monday for monitoring, though I am sure that will be a quick trip, and then back home. I can't race against time any longer. I'm just going to have faith and trust that all that happens next is what is meant to be. All I can do is breathe.

2 June 2012

Despite my protestations of breathing and calmness yesterday, I was actually feeling rather bad. As humans we want to control everything and my circumstances were not allowing that, I was making a show of being positive but perhaps not really digging it deep down.

Between then and now I dreamt I was baking cakes for my friend Roisin's birthday. I woke with an urge to enact some actual cake baking and I suddenly feel ridiculously happy. I spent half an hour on the phone to Roisin and it helped me not only shift my perspective but also cheered me up immensely. Instead of sullenly breathing myself around the house I'm having some fun. I've declared Molly cat a fan of Michael Jackson, sang his hits to her and now I'm searching recipes for cakes whilst introducing baby bump to the musical styling of Queen, Loving it.

I'm so lucky. Yeah, baby is taking some time to brew, but so what? I live in a free country, I have food in the cupboards, my prime minister has not issued a fatwa against me, I have entertainment coming out of my ears, and I have choices about everything. I can make cake on a whim and eat it or throw it all over the garden should I wish. I am as free as I want to be. The only prison is my own mind.

So I've found the key and I've let myself out. I'm going to bake cakes and maybe plant some stuff in the garden. After that I may read a magazine in the bath using my hot water that I'm so lucky to have piped right into my house.

As to the whole baby debacle, well she comes when she comes. My plans of natural birthing at a birthing centre are lovely, but they may not happen. I don't even care right now. If I go into labor I'm tempted to throw off my own plans and go to the local hospital if the birthing pool is free. Not sure why, possibly that's what my intuition wants. Whatever, whatever, whatever. I need to make cakes.

3 June 2012

Yesterday was lovely, I was in a fabulous mood. I made cakes, chocolate cake and carrot cake. I was pretty much upright and busy all day. Today the weather is grey and grumpy and I feel a little more fed up. I have been in town, wandered around and enjoyed a hot chocolate with marshmallows and lashings of cream. I'm back at home now with a less calorific raspberry leaf tea in front of me to stimulate my uterus. I'm also attempting nipple stimulation using my breast pump. Apparently this can be a very effective means of inducing labor. I have used the breast pump for about five minutes on each boob. Indeed this was made more entertaining by the fact I actually produced milk! The whole thing gave me a giggle and has put me in a better frame of mind. Plus, since doing it I do feel a lot more active in my belly and pelvis, which could mean either everything or nothing! However, I've concluded that nipple stimulation may be the way forward, it really is not as salacious as it sounds. Plus with nipple stimulating a dose of happy hormones have been released and this is better than a slap in the face. Boobs ahoy!

...My great boob mood didn't last. Had a random and unexpected fit of crying about the possibility of being induced. I'm so saddened even at the thought that I may be induced. I can cope with losing the potential naturalness of birth. What worries me is losing the peacefulness of birth. I want Poppyseed to come into the world in a calm, beautiful way. I'd planned that even down to the fake electric candles. Any step towards induction puts all that in jeopardy. So I had a cry about it. James was lovely and patient. He knows how important this is to me and he listened and said the right things, then he made me laugh with some daft comment. James also spoke a lot about why induction might be alright and the fact I was being a bit too negative. It all helped, he is my angel. I'm so lucky to have him.

Tomorrow morning I was supposed to be having the induction. Because I refused it, I agreed to go and be monitored instead. Fingers crossed that goes well and I get to leave and hopefully have my natural birth. I guess I'll ask again for a membrane sweep tomorrow. I'll try anything to avoid induction.

Dear Poppyseed,
Wherever your little soul is can you please call her in. We really love you and want to meet you soon. I think it's fair to say that even though we have not yet met you, we do already miss you. We want to bring you home gorgeous lady. See you super soon I hope.

Love,
Mummy.

4 June 2012
What a day. Woke up and went to the hospital at eight in the morning for monitoring. I was still too tight in the cervix for a sweep and I was encouraged by a doctor to have an induction by being told what danger I'm putting my baby in. I think that he was drafted in for the sole purpose of making me feel bad enough to agree. The pressure was immense. I agreed. I felt rushed, confused and a whole lot gutted. But when they start throwing statistics at you, it's so hard. I know there are two sides to the statistics story. I know what he is telling me is one very specific version of a much bigger picture. But right now, in a hospital, I can only see the version being presented to me. It was too hard.

We came home to get all my stuff and went back to hospital. I was monitored again for hours, strapped to a bed, bored, tired, stressed. Nothing moved, nothing really happened. Then it was time to start the induction…

Induction is a three-stage process. Hopefully the first stage is enough to get things started. But if after 24 hours labour hasn't started, then a further process is done that takes six hours. After that waters may be broken. Then if that still doesn't work then you are strapped to a bed with monitors, and injected with a drip that is pretty much guaranteed to bring on labor. If that doesn't work, then I guess Caesarean Section is the last resort left.

Just as they were literally about to start stage one and put a chemical pessary in me, the midwife informed me that I was now one centimeter dilated. That morning they'd said that there was no chance I'd dilate at all... At this stage I took the chance to stop the induction before it started and asked for a sweep instead. Two sweeps later and I am back home for the night chemical free.

I have, it seems, avoided chemical induction...for now. My cervix is my hero and thank god I spoke up and stopped that induction with literally seconds to spare. I am my own hero too.

It's been a bittersweet long, long day. Tears have been shed when I thought I was waving bye to my natural birth. James was so upset too because our hypnobirthing or birth preparations didn't prepare him for any of this. We have been blinkered in our approach. We have been so wrapped up in positive thinking, and envisioning the perfect birth, that none of this was ever an option. James is supposed to be looking after me, massaging me in a tub of water with twinkly music as accompaniment, whilst I om and ahh and meditate. But now he has had to take a back seat, it is my body being offered new options and only I can really make the choices. I can tell that he feels lost in this new plethora of serious medical information.

I've felt terrified at the implications of submitting to a chemical induction all day. But I've felt my power return when my cervix opened against all odds and now I'm just so relieved to be back home. I've seen two sides to the medical approach. The scary authoritative side that guilts you into following the guidelines and makes you think the very worst. But as I was leaving this evening, I saw the other side; a midwife cornered me and told me I have a choice, and that I still have some time on my hands. She is a midwife who knows a thing or two about Hypno/natural birthing and who has seen it in action. Her words were a little blessing.

Now it's time to relax and wait to see if the sweeps help get this baby show on the road. We didn't leave the hospital till about eight, I was there twelve hours. It's time to sleep, and then I'm back there again in the morning. At least by now they know who I am and what it is I'm trying to achieve. I've made that much very clear.

5 June 2012

The sweeps didn't work. I thought they were going to. In the night I had a lot of cramps, and I had a 'bloody show' on one of my toilet trips. I was so hopeful. But I woke up feeling normal, no pain, no gain… Came back to hospital this morning for more monitoring, hoping that it would be much quicker today. I left James at home to clean up as I was positive that it would be a quick visit. I asked my dad and stepmum Aileen to pick me up and take me, they heartily agreed. We sat around in the monitoring room having a good old chat, it was nice, for a while. I thought I'd be half a day maximum but, because of some issues with baby's heart rate dropping it seems, I have, yet again, agreed to be induced. Apparently the heart rate dropping can be a sign of distress. Part of me knows there is nothing wrong with my child. Call me daft but I know it.

At one point I asked everyone to leave so I could be as relaxed as possible. I listened to my hypnobirthing meditations and I chilled. The heart rate got better. But the previous drops were sufficient for the midwife to ask a doctor to come in, and I was given another lecture on the dangers of waiting. And so it seems

I am, again, to be induced.

I can't really remember what happened during the rest of the day. James was called and arrived. My Mum and Bev broke into the partner's waiting room. They thought I was ignoring them, but nobody told me they were there. I don't remember the induction itself. It's all a blur. After I'd had the induction pessary put in James and I went for a walk. We even tried to call in on his grandma as we walked past her house. We walked too far and had to call the TV crew to come pick us up because I started having some serious pains. My Mum brought an artillery of food for us, which was much needed as the hospital food was not exactly amazing. I was, for a time, given a room to myself, then it was taken away and I was on a shared ward. James had to leave in the evening...

It's now 10.50pm and I've been here since about 8am. There is one poor woman crying and pleading to be taken off a monitoring machine. She is saying it is making her feel worse, making her stressed, and this therefore is bad for her and for baby. Very reasonable logic. But having been strapped to a machine all day long, I also know that they will not remove her. The machines, whilst oppressive, save lives.

Prior to that, one other gal nearly gave birth outside the curtains that block me off from all the screaming women. Another woman was on her phone to her mother begging her to come be with her as she gave birth. From what I could tell her mum was refusing. I don't have that problem. My Mum, James's mum and my Dad and my step-mum Ailz have all been here since yesterday. All impatiently waiting and worrying and hoping... I'm lucky. Unfortunately I haven't really seen them. I've been strapped to machines. But I know they are here, somewhere.

Poppyseed's heartbeat has been normal ever since the monitoring where it kept dropping, but I'm in this thing now for the long haul. Now that I have a pessary in me, I have to wait 24 hours, unless I go into labor sooner.

I'm just trying to chill out, but my butt and undercarriage is aching like hell. I'm needing the toilet often, and it hurts like crazy to go. Not fun. I was a little dilated this morning so hopefully this first induction will work without resorting to any further drugs. Whilst the bringing on of labor will by no means be natural. The labor itself, once properly started, should be normal and without the requirement for any further drugs. I may even get to still use the birthing pool. I can refuse pain relief too of course. I'll make the most of this situation come hell or high water.

As I mentioned, all the grandparents have been here today. It's nice to be so supported. Though my Mum and Bev were removed from the ward for causing a nuisance, which at least gave me and James a giggle. They were all here before I even went into labor; I find it sweet and funny. The film crew are about also, which proves a nice distraction. They have a great opportunity to now capture me make up free, lank haired, white faced and moaning. After months of being a glam mum-to-be, dressing up my bump and accessorizing perfectly, they now get the real me. No, they don't actually, they get the shabby, pale, exhausted me. Really though, I am past caring. I hope Miss Poppyseed soon finds a way out to her adoring public.

As for induction. I feel I'm caught somewhere between an alternative health mafia and a medical mafia. They both mean well, but they have extremely different thoughts on achieving the same goal – a healthy, happy baby. I've had to question a great deal and dig into my own intuition. In the end it's all about the baby. I've made every final decision with her welfare as the end goal. When I was told that her heart was not behaving as it should there was little else I could, or wanted to do. So I embraced an induction. I'm getting to be cool with this now. Sort of…

6 June 2012

Last night I felt I was in labor all night. Besides that I barely slept for all the screaming and crying going on. Horrific. It was a long, slow night. No one spoke to me and people were in and out having babies whilst I just lay on my bed suffering. My whole undercarriage hurts, my stomach is having contractions, and yet they won't check this out until later…

…24 hours later, I've been checked. Nothing. I'm two centimeters dilated. What the hell those pains have been about I'll never know. I don't know what happens next? I've struggled to get answers. I'm getting distressed. I want to go home. The food here is crap. Nobody medical has spoken to me all day. James and Roisin are here, they are keeping me upbeat, I can see James is flagging though as much as me. Claire and Donovan are here, not even filming all the time, just being good company. We don't want me to be here. We want me to be at home. I bumped into my midwife Jo from the local doctors surgery, I sent her off to get information. This helped, she is sweet…

…I have been given a six-hour induction pessary. Damn we are on the second stage now. If this works I still have the option of a natural-ish birth. I can still use the birth pool. I can avoid the full on chemical drip that means I'm stuck on a bed being monitored and unable to move. James has had to go home. Claire from the film crew, snuck me a pizza in after visiting hours. I can't tell you how happy this makes me.

I need to sleep. I'm so afraid of waking up in pain and James not being here. This is not how this was supposed to go. If I go into labor he should be here, with me, holding my hand. But that is what I'm facing. Pizza is my only solace. At least tonight it seems quieter here…

…I need to get out of here. Two failed induction attempts, twenty-four hours of agony later and six hours of nothing and I'm sick of it. This baby is not for shifting, I feel like I've been fobbed off and ignored. I'm such low priority I may as well just grow facial hair and call myself a bloke. I thought my baby was in trouble, but I'm hardly on anyone's priority list! It's 2.30am and I've woken up with not an ounce of pain. I want pain! I want labor. I want these attempts to work. But they haven't, and I'm sad and lonely and I want to go home.

I was told with the last lot of drugs that I could have a 24-hour break. I want a 24-hour break, this place is a joke and I'm sick of it. I'm not taking Poppyseed to the next stage of drips and potentially me having surgery. Not when there is no medical reason whatsoever. It's been a fun little NHS break, but I've had enough. Well and truly had enough, this child deserves better. I deserve better. I WANT OUT!

Spoke with James and he is so helpless, bless him. He told me to come home; he could hear the hurting in my voice. I agreed and then I spoke with my current midwife (they change constantly) and attempted to leave. I told her I was getting in a taxi and going home. She however talked me round and I stayed in hospital.

...I slept amazingly and feel a lot better than I did at 3am this morning. Feeling emotional about meeting Poppyseed. In that respect, I feel different. Every day I've been very stressed, tired, scared but today I have a feeling I will be meeting my daughter. When she is here I want to bundle her in my arms and take her on holiday because she deserves it. Maybe I can take her with James to the seaside, in a week or so. I love her so much, I hope today is the day.

Dear Poppyseed,
Mummy is having a hard time getting you into this world. But I suspect its 'cos you aren't yet ready. Silly old hospital has tried to rush us. I feel closer to you today so maybe that's a sign. Maybe next week we can go to the seaside together. I can't wait for

cuddle time with you. You are so beautiful. I love you darling so let's get this show on the road home, my little baby angel darling.

Love

Mummy

7 June 2012

Another day, another procedure, more decisions, more internal fighting for a natural birth. First thing this morning a Doctor broke my waters and gave me two hours to go into labor naturally before more induction occurred. I sat there waiting for my waters to actually start coming out. I was being interviewed on camera about how I felt. I laughed about something. This started a flood down below. I laughed more, more flooding. I got in hysterics, laughing my daft little head off. Flooding, flooding, flooding. James and the crew were laughing too because they knew from my face what was going on under the bed covers. Thank goodness they sit you on giant pads! During the hysteria that followed I knocked my monitoring equipment awry – yes I am still strapped up. Had a midwife come and tell me to stop laughing as it was moving the monitors. It felt like I had been told off at school and so then I got the giggles. No laughing in the birthing ward people. Screaming and crying are acceptable, but god forbid anyone laughs!

More hilarity as I tried to get dressed with a constant drip, gush, drip of amniotic fluid. I destroyed a rainforest of tissues trying to keep up. James and I needed this little laugh. Amniotic fluid, the gift that just keeps on giving!

After two hours nothing had happened in terms of going into labor. Yet still determined to have some kind of natural birth I refused the induction till evening. This was a stressful decision but I felt powerfully that I needed more time. I needed to try to avoid the chemical drip induction so that I could enact some of my birthing plan. It was a last ditch attempt at grasping some power back. As ever, throughout this whole mess, I was just determined to claw back some kind of natural ending.

James and I tried to distract ourselves and get baby moving. We walked and waked round the hospital corridors, we stimulated nipples with a breast pump. I went to the hospital chapel and prayed. As I was sat in the chapel, I got an automated message from the pregnancy application on my phone. Quite pertinently it said, 'I am confident that my birthing will happen at the right time for my baby.' This set me off in floods of tears. I guess I interpret it as meaning that whatever happens, it is right. Given the set of events that followed this makes a reassuring thought.

The Birth Story.

What happened next was that at about two in the afternoon I caved in to the medical model and it's demands for induction. I had spoken with my Doula Mia, her words buoyed me up for a while but then I realized how extremely tired James and I were. I decided to stop waiting and just do what I was advised. There was nothing left to fight for. The fight was killing us both. We couldn't walk away at this stage and choose to wait. The only power left to me was the miniscule power of just getting on with it and having a baby. The inevitability of induction was here and now.

By now I knew in my heart I wouldn't go into labor myself, waiting was a mugs game and so forward to the drip it was. Because James and I were both so drained we also decided we needed a third party to act as a breath of fresh air. So at this, Roisin was re-invited to be a birth partner via James making a tearful phone call requesting her attendance. She attended nearly immediately and we went full scale ahead into the chemical induction procedure.

This involved being hooked up to a chemical drip that would bring on contractions and would slowly be turned up to make the contractions stronger.

Gone are the fluffy 'surges' of hypnobirthing, we were embarked on a full-scale medical intervention. I couldn't eat, I couldn't drink. This was made worse by the fact my Mum had again brought a whole load of yummy looking food for us to chow down on. So I watched James and Roisin have a birthing picnic instead! Worse than that though, I just really wanted a cup of tea. No such luck. I had to wee in a cardboard chamber pot and I was hooked up to a number of wires for monitoring as well as a second fluid drip to keep me hydrated. Everything I dreamed of was out the window. But me being me, I figured that this must be what was meant to happen as it so clearly was what was happening. You can't argue with fate. I tried, I failed. So rather than rail against what was happening I embraced it as wholeheartedly as I knew how.

For the first few hours I managed the contractions using hypnobirthing techniques, just my breathing and occasional meditation. We had music playing and I could still use my essential oils, so at least the room smelt good. We managed to whip up a relaxed friendly atmosphere. We were actually having fun. Even when the contractions were challenging, it was a jovial, fun affair. I meditated, I listened to my hypnobirthing affirmations. It felt good. That much of my birth plans I could still enact. A midwife and a student midwife accompanied us and at times Claire was there too, sometimes filming, sometime just chatting. It was going rather well.

...But then the induction drug got turned up a notch and I nearly immediately lost the ability to cope. Breathing and visualization felt wholly useless against the onslaught of five painful rolling contractions per ten minutes. The pain very quickly became extreme and the facets of hypnobirthing were left lolling around uselessly in the dust. I've since been told that the chemical induction is 'evil' in terms of pain, whilst hypno-birthing may help a woman handle a natural birth, it lost its efficacy when challenged by this medically-enforced labor.

I was not in a good place. I felt I was being torn apart, and so suddenly. Panic was rising and I felt truly scared. You know when you see women on TV saying 'I can't do it', well that was pretty much how I felt. There was no let up between contractions. This was not how it was supposed to be. It was not the gentle hum of contraction followed by break, followed by cup of tea that I had visualized. The contractions did not get progressively stronger, so that I could find ways to 'be' with them. They just got strong. Full stop. It was constant, relentless, searing pain.

So strapped up to the monitor, stuck on my back on a bed, I desperately decided to try gas and air to regain some sense of control. For a few moments this was terrific. At first it amused me how 'high' I felt. I thought I was a comedian all of a sudden and took great pleasure in announcing to the room, in a bizarre deep voice that seemed to come with the gas and air, that I felt so 'fucking high'. Nice language, momma! I then pointedly looked into the camera, and retorted, that I had never smoked marijuana, raised eyebrow, and cheeky grin. It was funny because it was so unexpected. James said I came out with a few hilarious comments, but he has since forgotten them all. So have I. Because once those few jokes had come out of my mouth, I realized that whilst I may feel high as a kite, this was not a good trip.

The high did not in any respect outweigh the pain. Indeed I felt totally lost and terrified that I could no longer communicate with James and Roisin, or anyone else, because of the effects of the gas and air. Everything went trippy, I was stuck in my head and I couldn't interact with the room. Yet the pain was still there. Gas and air did not give me control, it made me lose the remnants of it that I had left. In my memory this went on maybe half an hour or so. James tells me it was more like two hours and that he came and went from the room, at one point having something to eat.

I don't remember this part very well. Any of this could have happened at any time, I simply don't know. I remember pertinent points. But I don't have any kind of timeline in my memory. Indeed James has told me that I have the timeline all messed up and confused, but that is how it is, so I guess that is how I will report it here.

I remember seeing desperation and fear on James and Roisin's faces. At some point Roisin worked her way to my side and was stroking my head, which was nice. I don't know how she got there. At another point I heard James crying and he jokes now about how rude I was to him in requesting him to stop crying. He was suffering alongside me, but I couldn't cope with his tears, it was one thing too much. I apparently I told him to stop crying, because how was I supposed to cope when he was cracking up, I think I did so with all the politeness I could muster... I remember planning it in my head very carefully. What I said was direct and straight to the point. I needed him to pull it together. I think I hurt his feelings, but I had a good point, I needed him to cope, and he obeyed, so I got what I needed! I didn't mean to be a bitch but he was breaking my heart. Which was too much to bear alongside the pain.

At some point, a midwife angel drifted in and told me that she too had wanted a natural 'sit and squat' birth, but that she had been induced and that it was hard for her as well. She told me I had done well coping so far, but that I should consider my pain relief options. She laid them out for me. I wasn't willing to commit, even in spite of the agony, so instead we had a look at how far I had progressed. If I was ten centimeters then great, we could get on with birth, if I was much less, then pain relief might be needed.

They checked me over and I was still only two centimeters

dilated, after all those hours and all that pain... I decided to have an epidural, as it was the one thing that would not directly affect the baby. James was out of the room when I chose this. He was so confused when he came back in, thinking it had been forced upon me. But no. I needed it. I wanted it. There was no two ways around it. I was in agony and the one thing I thought I would never ever have, an epidural, I needed and I needed it now.

I was still sucking on the gas and air like a crazy woman when the anesthetist arrived. Frustratingly, he had to ask me lots of questions, and I may even have had to sign something. By this point I was more or less begging him to hurry up. I am sure I was probably in tears or near to it. I know I was likely grunting and moaning. I was 'that' woman, the one I swore I wouldn't be. The one I hoped hypnobirthing would help me avoid. Though I did not scream, and trust me, I spent several days on the labor ward, there is a whole lotta screaming going on! It was hell; I've never felt more desperate. I just wanted some semblance of peace back. I didn't want to bring baby into the world in this way, panicked and in desperate pain.

The epidural brought me back to life. Though the gas and air affected my realization that the epidural had actually worked. I had become so dependent on it, even though I hated it, I was sucking on that pipe like mad, even when all the people in the room were telling me I was no longer in pain. That information took a while to sink in. Poor James was trying to give me a count down as to when the epidural would work, and I snapped at him to stop telling me times. I remember him saying 'only 20 minutes'. And I remember thinking 'Only! Only!' There is no 'only' about a whole twenty minutes when you are feeling like that. Poor bloke!

I also accused James of looking at things over my shoulder and pulling faces. He was apparently looking at the machine that showed contractions that were practically off the chart they were so strong. All I could see was him looking past me at something unknown. I guess I took exception to this.

Having felt lost in some weird trippy wilderness, the epidural gave us back peace. It was amazing. It was perfect. It was not what I wanted, but it gave me what I desired. I was myself again and poor James was no longer the brunt of my pain-induced temper!

From here on in, it was a long night. I could still feel the massive pressure of the contractions despite the epidural, but the sharp pain was gone. Towards the end it came back, but was manageable. Roisin felt poorly and had to leave at about one in the morning, and James went for a sleep at one point. I was alone with the midwives for some hours, and happily they were lovely and friendly, and young too.

I tried to rest, but this was hampered by their concerns. Baby's heartbeat kept dropping after each contraction and my temperature was raised. At one point, I remember feeling really, really sick, though I never vomited. I think it passed when I had some water. In spite of all this, I knew everything would be okay. Even when they were drafting in doctors and talking of potential Caesarean sections, I knew baby was fine, and that I would be too.

Probably around 2am I had the urge to push. But it was not until they checked me at around 4am that they discovered I was fully dilated. I believe I had been for some time.

We waited an hour and then the pushing began in earnest. Again threats of Caesarean Section were made. So I tried to push harder. The epidural made it difficult to push and the contractions were not as strong as they had been. I pushed for nearly an hour and a half. Again this was down to me asking for more time, still trying so hard to avoid less natural options. I wanted to do it myself. I really did. I still had that fighting spirit even after everything.

My room felt crowded with women. In my memory, there were about eight of them all willing me to push, with a lovely

Indian doctor being the most vocal of them all. I also remember how pretty all the midwifes were. It was like a glamorous hospital drama shoot, not a gritty real life hospital room in middle England. Glamorous except for me, I'm sure I looked like hell. So in front of all these gorgeous girls, I had my legs spread and was doing my best to 'push, push, push, push' for my team of cheerleaders!

The pushing didn't work. The forceps were brought in. From here on in it was pretty definite I would meet my girl in a few pushes and pull's time. James took his place at my head and held my hand tight (probably – I don't really remember). The forceps looked like giant salad spoons and thank god that epidural was effective, because having them inserted would not have been pleasant. I was given an episiotomy too, one more thing on the list of things I didn't want. Really though I couldn't care less anymore. Better be cut than to tear due to those damned salad spoons.

So the Doctor pulled and I pushed as much as I could. We stalled between contractions and maybe Poppyseed's head was out, maybe it wasn't. It felt like a long wait, James said it was quick. Then that final contraction and bang...

There she was. There she was. There she was.

Tiny, tired and blue on my bare chest. Daddy nearly fainted. I grabbed his hand and we both touched her. Then she was gone. Whisked off and I don't know why, because she hadn't cried? They wanted her to cry. The cord must have been cut by unknown hands, not by James. I was given an injection. The doctor held up my placenta as if from nowhere, a massive slab of meat, then it was gone. That was supposed to happen naturally? She was supposed to stay on my chest… Was everything okay? A light was shining on her and I asked them, please turn that off. They did. And all the while my eyes; my eyes were on Poppyseed pinking up on a table just a few meters away.

Then she was back. And she didn't cry. Not at all. Why should she? But she was alert and she saw me and I saw her, she kept blinking, and Daddy saw her and she saw Daddy. Sam Cooke was playing in the background. It was the break of dawn. I was half naked and she took to my breast and her eyes, bruised from the forceps sparkled. And she didn't cry, but she was alert. And we held her. And we kissed her. And she didn't cry all day, but she was so alert. And she had a flock of brown hair on her little bruised head. And she was beautiful. And she looked like Daddy. And we loved her forevermore.

Dear Ivy Belle
I can't be left alone with you. Whenever I am, I end up flooded by tears of happiness. I'm scared I may drown us both. I've never experienced a feeling like this, you are everything. You are my heart and my soul. I never want to leave you. I never want to be apart from you. You are the most incredible, perfect, beautiful person I've ever known, even when you are crying. I'm obsessed, fanatical, desperately crazily in love. You have been here four days and they have been the most precious, wonderful days I've ever known.

I thought this letter would be easy to write. But I'm struggling as no one has yet invented the words I need to describe my love for you. Here are the few that nearly hit the spot – sacred, profound, earth shattering, life changing, beautiful, incredible, astounding, transformative, joyous, ecstatic, stunning.

My love for you is a whole new experience of being. All else drops away and you stand at the centre of all life. Of all creation. I don't mean you to feel any pressure by any of this either; whatever you do or become in life all of this always applies forever and ever. Wherever you go, whoever you are, no matter how many mistakes you make, or successes you achieve all of the above is always the fresh and newest truth.

You can do no wrong, not really because whatever you do will see me at your side supporting, helping, loving, caring… If I ever become a worrying mother just know that at the heart of it sits the purest thing, the most powerful thing, the deepest love ever known, the love of a momma for her Poppyseed.

Ivy Belle, you are my left, right, up and down. You are my inside and out my truest and my true, my pink to blue. You are my new black, my sunset and rise. Everything that was remotely soulful in my life pales in comparison to your beautiful eyes.

I'm all shook up sweet, sweet girl and you are the roller coaster of love causing it, every love song ever written now applies to you. Every poem, every perfect moment, every romance, every deep belly laugh, every scrap of affection, every heartache and break and lovelorn fantasy. Tie all these emotions up, bundle them in one person and this is somewhere close to how I feel.

My baby Belle bottom, momma is no doubt making you blush. I love you, simple and concise and eternally. You are carried at my heart as you were all day yesterday and a good chunk of last night, and that is where you will stay forever… Deep in my chest, implanted in my heart, carried on my breath, first before all things.

Always and forever,
Your Momma Alice

Soulful Momma Resources, as mentioned by Alice

The Mother Magazine www.themothermagazine.co.uk

Hypnobirthing, The Mongan Method, The breakthrough approach to safer, easier, comfortable birthing, Marie Mongan, 2007, Souvenir Press

Mia Scotland (Doula and Hypnobirthing) Your Birth Right - www.yourbirthright.co.uk/

Healthy Pregnancy In A Box, Annie Lawler www.breathing-spacetherapies.co.uk

Ina May's Guide to Childbirth, Ina May Gaskin, Ebury Digital, 9 June 2010

My Pregnancy Today - Phone Application from Baby Centre – www.babycentre.co.uk

The Hypnobirthing Centre with Katherine Graves – Phone Application – www.hypnobirthingcentre.co.uk

The Complete Pregnancy Workout Boxed Set Including Yoga, Pilates, Fitness and Postnatal, Acacia DVD

Your Pregnancy Bible, Consulting Editor Dr Annie Deans, Carroll and Brown Publishers Limited, 2003

And when baby is here Alice LOVES...

Ask Dr Sears, A Trusted resource for Parents www.askdrsears.com

Kellymom Parenting and Breastfeeding www.kellymom.com

Other Books by Alice Grist

The High Heeled Guide to Enlightenment

The High Heeled Guide to Enlightenment is the must have book for females who are looking to connect to something other than their internet provider! Alice Grist jumps stilettos first into all things spiritual and conjures up an entertaining, witty and honest account of her search for Enlightenment. The High Heeled Guide brings an understanding of alternative spirituality to a new audience. It is spirituality for the sexy socialite, enlightenment for the lipgloss dependent and a crash course in serenity for the yummy mummy! Veering between the wildly faddish and fashionable to the freakier and less familiar, the High Heeled Guide sheds a pink and intelligent spotlight upon a diverse collection of spiritual options that well suit the modern Woman. An intriguing, informative and hilarious read for any Woman who knows deep in her worn down sole that there is more to life than cars, careers, kids and cocktails.

The High Heeled Guide to Spiritual Living (Prediction Magazine Best Book Award)

The High Heeled Guide to Spiritual Living is a passionate, fiery and funny account that shows how to bring the deliciously soulful into modern life. It demonstrates how in a world overrun by rampant egos, consumerism and celebrity you can spiritualize your sanity and revamp your life for the benefit of your soul, and all with a side dish of feisty feminine panache! The High Heeled Guide to Spiritual Living discloses delicious spiritual secrets and intimately reveals how to easily manifest these mysteries into your reality. A definitive guide for anyone who desires a truly spiritual life.

Follow Alice's continued journey as a Soulful Momma here: www.alicegrist.co.uk

Soul Rocks is a fresh list that takes the search for soul and spirit mainstream. Chick-lit, young adult, cult, fashionable fiction & non-fiction with a fierce twist